# AMAZING THINGS
# YOU DON'T KNOW
## ABOUT YOUR OWN BODY

As far as I could perfunctorily verify (limited as I was by the dual restraints of time and sustainable enthusiasm), located within are honest to goodness true facts. But let's face it, with a book fairly bristling with information like this one, it is slightly possible that a small (bordering on paltry) number of the entries inside might be slightly less than 100% accurate. Although the odds of such are laughingly small, I urge that you resist making any important medical decisions based on the information contained herein, within, or inside.* In fact, on the off-chance that you do encounter a suspect fact or figure, your assignment is to immediately e-mail** me substantiated information to the contrary. Who knows, this and/or a generous contribution of other "amazing things" uncovered, or even discovered by you, may find an honored place within subsequent issues of this already inspirational tome.

* attempt at legalese
** atydkayob@hotmail.com

ISBN: 1-4392-2119-7
ISBN-13: 9781439221198

Visit www.booksurge.com to order additional copies.

# AMAZING THINGS

# YOU
# DON'T
# KNOW

## ABOUT

# YOUR OWN BODY

(Proof That Your Body is Far More Wonderful
Than it Looked in the Mirror This Morning)

BY **MIKE BELL**

**P**repare to be dazzled by your own incredible body. The amazing facts and figures inside this book describing you and your giblets, come from literally days of in-depth research into textbooks and Internet sites, as well as the systematic badgering of students, colleagues, and ex-friends, (to all of which and whom I express my heartfelt gratitude).

# INDEX

# The Digestive System

Think about all of the culinary question marks you've casually dumped into your mouth over the years. Your digestive system is stuck with the daunting task of making something useful out of it all. Basically a 20–30 foot tube (depending on whether you're alive or not at measuring time), snaking its way through your body, the digestive plumbing inside you has the absolutely amazing ability to: a) break down meals ranging from tuna fish to Twinkies into the precise raw materials that your body needs to grow, perform, and repair itself; b) eliminate the small percentage of stuff that it can't break down (because most of us would just hate having to chew our cud—even if we could) and, c) recycle almost all of the water contained in that tuna/Twinkie meal and make it available for dozens of bodily processes (including manufacturing the very juices needed to help digest your next dose of Pepto Bismol). Your amazing digestive system performs this selective food processing both chemically (with digestive enzymes) and mechanically (chews, churns, and chugs), and most of the time without complaint. If, however, it does have a problem, we invariably hear about it.

**1. The average human produces 25,000 quarts of spit in a lifetime (we anatomists prefer the term "saliva").**

* That's enough to fill the average-sized backyard swimming pool half way to the top.

**2. All of the 50 species of *beneficial* bacteria in your large intestines (colon), about 100 trillion of them, would just about fill a coffee mug. They are so small that the individual bacteria in your colon outnumber the total number of cells in your body by about 2 to 1.**

* Up to 40% of our feces (rhymes with "oop") can be composed of these rapidly producing "beneficial flora," and they are a large part of the reason why your fecal material tends to be brown no matter how colorful your meal was.

* On average, each of us produces a little more than 300 pounds of fecal "material" per year (about the weight of 3 runway models-sorry)

**3. Death occurs in a starving person in a matter of weeks, while a person can die from sleep deprivation in about 10 days (that's why having a newborn in the house can be both a joyous and near-death experience).**

**4. In the U.S., 200,000 appendectomies are performed every year. It is estimated that 40,000 of these are performed on patients who turned out *not* to have appendicitis (a diseased appendix).**

* P.S.: It is reported that an average of 16 Canadians have their appendixes removed unnecessarily *every day.*

**5. In the good ol' days, every time you licked a stamp you consumed approximately 1/10 of a calorie (Kcal). Don't worry, though. If you went on a stamp-licking frenzy today, it would take about 35,000 stamp-lickings for you to gain one pound of body weight (*not* factoring in the caloric expenditure required to lick them in the first place, *and* the calories generated digesting the small but significant amounts of animal by-product consumed during the ordeal).**

**6. During the average lifetime, an American consumes between 30 and 50 *tons* of food (about 600 times your weight—if you weigh between 100 and 167 pounds).**

* That's about the weight of 6 medium sized elephants (*Loxodonta Africana*).

---

**7. During your lifetime, you spend an average total of 4 years simply engaged in the act of eating food.**

**8. At birth, we each have 52 developing teeth buried in our gums. The first batch to emerge, the 20 "baby" teeth (deciduous), are preparing to "erupt" as they are needed. Later, we "lower" 32 permanent teeth, but many of us have up to 4 of them, the ones we call "wisdom teeth," removed.**

**9. The average person (yes, including beauty queens) releases one quart of flatulence (intestinal gas—rhymes with "carts") per day, in 10 to 15 "installments." Most of this gas is due to swallowed air during eating (we swallow an average of 300 times during dinner, and once a minute during the rest of the day). The rest is due to fermentation of undigested food.**

* By the way: If you collected all of the gas an average human passes over 6 years and 9 months, and then ignited it, the resultant explosion would contain energy approaching that of a one megaton atomic bomb (I imagine that the fatalities would also be comparable).

---

*Because of pressure, scuba divers reportedly cannot pass gas at depths of 33 feet or more. (I am sure our aquatic friends appreciate that fact)

---

**10. The digestive tract is a thirty-foot tube through your body—about the length of the average size school bus.**

* Cited digestive tube (alimentary canal) lengths vary, not only because of the size of the human measured, but because the length of the tube varies quite a bit depending on whether the subject is living (shorter) or dead (longer).

---

\* In case you were wondering; the digestive system of a horse is about 90 feet long—(It's also interesting that if a horse swallows something horrible, it can't vomit like you and I can).

## 11. Your stomach produces a completely new lining every 2–3 days, or it would digest itself.

\* 500,000 stomach lining cells die and must be replaced *every minute* because *35 million* secreting glands there produce an acid (hydrochloric) stronger than battery acid (pH of 1-2), and powerful enough to dissolve a razor blade in 4 days. Mucous glands, located right next to the acid-producing ones, secrete a mucus that does its best to protect the lining from destruction.

## 12. Our stomach produces about one gallon of these gastric juices every day.

## 13. The main reason for our own odoriferous (stinky) fecal material (see #2) are foul elements (indole and scatole) produced by the 400 species of bacteria inside of you. This is also why your armpits smell, by the way.

## 14. Our digestive system is very efficient at extracting and absorbing nutrients from the food we eat. Of all the food eaten on a daily basis, an average of only 2/3 pound leaves the body as feces, and in general, most of that comes from the indigestible parts of plant material (cellulose).

\* By the way: Cows can digest cellulose, but they have 4 stomachs (chambers) to do the job, *and* have to regurgitate and then chew their food again to boot (rumination). No thanks. I'll get my fiber some other way.

## 15. Your digestive system has two hormones that regulate your appetite. One (ghrelin) makes you feel hungry, and the other (leptin) tells your brain that your stomach is full.

## 16. During our lifetimes, we Americans consume an average of 12 pounds of food additives, and about one gallon of pesticides. Some of these chemicals tend to remain in your body "forever."

17. The average human consumes 70 insects (and 10 spiders) during the lifetime of even the most careful eating (although I suspect that the combined efforts of some 3rd world "epicureans," as well as a few upper-level college entomology courses, *may* kick the average up a bit).

18. During a typical year, we eat *our weight* in sugars (glucose, fructose, maltose, corn syrup, Sorbitol, saccharine, dextrose, molasses, honey, etc.).

19. When you blush, the lining of your stomach also turns red.

20. Digestion takes 10% of our daily energy requirements (70% is needed to operate other bodily processes, which leaves only 20% for all of your demanding physical activities).

21. In our lifetimes, we Americans consume an average of

➤ 8000 eggs,
➤ 6000 loaves of bread,
➤ ½ ton of cheese,
➤ 1000 gallons of milk (only 1/10 the amount of milk that the average cow can dispense" during its lifetime)
➤ a ton of fruit,
➤ 200 pounds of peanuts,
➤ 10,000 pounds of meat, including 200 chickens and 23 pigs,(in various forms),
➤ 406 gallons of ice cream,
➤ 600 sticks of chewing gum,
➤ 35,000 cookies, and
➤ 1610 pounds of pizza (about the weight of 4 Italian chefs—just kidding).

* By the way: In the U.S. alone, we consume an average of 357 slices of pizza, 600 hot dogs, and 7,000 Cokes—*per second* (that's about 1 1/2 acres of the pizza, 49 miles of hot dogs, and about 86 Olympic sized swimming pools full of Coke per day).

**22. Essential components of our digestive system are our 3 pairs of salivary glands, which secrete up to 2 pints of saliva each day. This juice not only lubricates our food for the trip through the 30 foot digestive tube, but contains an enzyme (ptyalin, or salivary amylase) which actually begins to digest starches while still in our mouth.**

\* You can check the effectiveness of those salivary enzymes by moistening a ball of white bread, putting it on a plate, and watching it dissolve into a puddle of sugars right before your eyes. Or try this: place back into the jar the spoon you just used to sample the baby food. Notice the clear layer of fluid that develops around the spoon? Yep, starch into sugar.

**23. The glasslike material (enamel) on the surface of your teeth is the hardest substance in the human body, and is about as hard as glass. Interestingly, the surface of your tooth is the only body part that cannot easily repair itself.**

**24. Some vitamins and minerals are absolutely essential for your health, and yet are needed in such small quantities that a *lifetime supply* of them would fill less than ½ a thimble.**

**25. The liver provides energy and raw materials for body repair. After a meal, this chemical factory acts as a manufacturer and supplier, as well as waste-disposal unit and chemical detoxifier. It is a protector, a regulator, and a facilitator of many bodily processes.**

**26. The liver has more than 500 distinct functions, some of which are essential for digesting the food we eat. It can continue to operate with the loss of as many as 80-90% of its cells through disease or injury. No machine (or combination of machines) in the world today could duplicate the many functions of your liver (in a package even thousands of times larger).**

**27. The liver (also discussed in the "immune" portion of this book) is made of 75,000 groups of identical cells (300 billion altogether); and unlike almost any other organ, has a double blood supply running through it.**

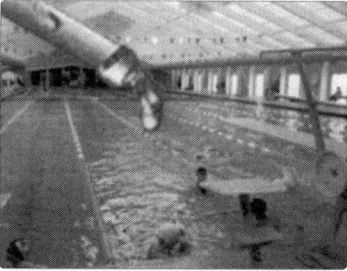

*How many is 300 Billion?: Almost 5 times the total number of people who have died during recorded history; the number of drops of water in 4 Olympic Swimming pools or, the number of Tootsie Rolls eaten every 2.2 years

28. The liver requires that about ¼ of the body's blood supply pass through it in order to perform its many functions. Blood flows through it at a rate of 1 ¾ pints every minute (about 1/6 of the flow rate through the heart itself).

29. More than 80% of the water (about 10 pints every day) contained in the food we are digesting (chyme) is filtered out by the colon (the last 6 feet of intestines), and is passed into the circulatory system for distribution.

30. If (for a variety of reasons) the food you eat speeds through the digestive system too quickly, the colon won't have time to absorb enough water from it, and you will experience diarrhea. If the food spends too much time there, you will suffer from constipation.

31. The people in Denmark eat an average of 29.5 pounds of chocolate per year. That's about one ton per Dane, per lifetime (Americans eat an average of 350 pounds of the wonderful stuff in a lifetime).

* But don't feel too outclassed. That's still a respectable equivalent of 3,733 Hershey candy bars each, for a total of 864,590 calories (equivalent to 24.7 pounds of body weight).

32. The macroscopic (visible) surface area of a set of human intestines is about 6 square feet, but if you include the microscopic projections (bumps) called villi which line last 11 feet of the small intestines (ileum), the surface area increases 250 *times*—to 1500 square feet (slightly less than the surface area of a volleyball court).

**33. The small intestines (duodenum, jejunum, and ileum) stretched out, are about 21 feet of the 30 foot intestinal tract; about the same length as a French horn (and except for the first few months of music lessons, producing far less pleasing sounds).**

\* In case you were wondering, the medical term for the "growly" noise your intestines make while digesting food is called BORBORYGMOS. (See the "FUN" vocabulary index.)

**34. The digestive system is so efficient at doing its job that most of the material in feces is made of cellulose (indigestible plant fiber). intestinal bacteria, lining tissue from the walls of the canal itself, and old bile (digestive juice made in the liver, which, combined with intestinal bacteria, accounts for the color). The amazing thing is that almost _all_ of the available nutrients in the food you swallow is processed, absorbed and then pushed into the circulatory system for distribution.**

**35. Each human tooth may have up to 55 _miles_ of microscopic canals in it—for the circulation of oxygen and nutrients to the tooth.**

**36. The average American consumes 3,757 Kcals (calories) daily. By contrast, the average caloric intake around the world is 2,474 calories per day. An American, reduced to that caloric intake level could lose (not necessarily all fat) about a pound every 3 days.**

\* Within the past 30 years, the average caloric intake, for Americans, has gone up 335 Kcals (calories) per day. Without factoring in physical activity, that figure alone would amount to a weight gain of about a pound of body weight every ten days.

\* To add perspective to the above, _9 million_ people starve to death in the world every year (one every 3.6 seconds), and 6 million of them are under age 5.

**37. If the amount of water in your body is reduced by one part in 100 (1%), you feel thirsty. With a loss of 10%, you are in danger of dying (of dehydration or heat stroke).**

**38. You will drink about 20,000 gallons of water during your lifetime;** enough to full 2 average sized swimming pools (no doubt much more if you are actually a swimmer).

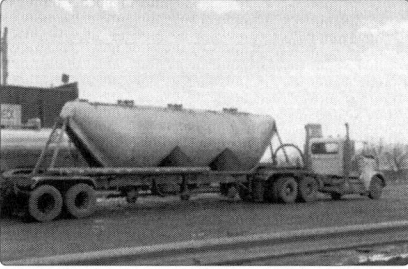

* 20,000 gallons is the amount held by three milk tanker trucks.

**39. The average human body contains 30 to 40 million fat cells, both on the inside, cushioning and supporting your giblets, and on the outside, "adorning" your body (and generating a variety of feelings about mirrors). These fat cells are filling up and emptying as your pant size changes.**

* The number of fat cells will remain constant throughout your life—unless you decide to slurp them out with liposuction, that is.

**40. We mammals have a growth factor in our mouths which make its cells the fastest healing tissue in the body.**

**41. The average stomach can hold just under 2 quarts of food, and in so doing can stretch up to 50 *times* its empty size.**

*On July 4th 2007, 230 pound American, Joey Chestnut cemented his place in "gurgitating" history by consuming 66 hot dogs (including buns) in 12 minutes. Takeru Kobayashi, the diminutive 131 pound Japanese eating phenomenon, had previously held the record for 5 consecutive years.

**42. If the beneficial bacteria in your colon ever found their way from the "tube through your body," which is the digestive system, and *into* your body via the circulatory system, death could easily be the result.**

**43. Before their first birthday, the average baby will have dribbled 255 pints of saliva (not to mention other bi-polar events).**

* 255 pints is about 32 gallons—enough to fill a fish tank 6 feet long, 3 feet high, and 2 feet wide (but don't expect even the toughest fish to survive in there for very long).

---

**44. One of the purposes of the uvula (the "hangy-down" thing from the roof of your mouth) is to swing up when you swallow which shuts off some of the passage to your nostrils. Otherwise, a small amount of liquid could dribble out of your nose with each swallow. Some anatomists feel that the uvula also signals the "trap door" (epiglottis) covering your breathing tube (trachea) to close when you swallow, to help prevent food from getting stuck in your airway.**

**45. Eating ice cream (actually anything cold will do) slows down and stops the digestion process until the "plumbing" warms up again.**

**46. When you become excited (say at a football game) your stomach muscles contract strongly, and the output of digestive juices triples (which is perhaps why stadium and theater food sells so well, even at those ridiculous prices).**

**47. In addition to the rhythmic, pulsating motion of the digestive tract (peristalsis) which pushes food (actually called "chyme" at this point) through, there is a swaying motion to the tract (the intestines are loosely connected to the abdominal wall). In fact, your suspended digestive tract sways back and forth an average of 10-15 times per minute.**

**48. The 6–10 inch long, dog-tongue-like pancreas produces 2 pints of Sodium Bicarbonate (baking soda) each day which helps neutralize the acids produced by your stomach. This amazing organ also produces insulin (unless you are diabetic) which helps regulate sugars. This makes the pancreas the only combination endocrine ("inside-secreting") and exocrine ("exo"=outside) gland in your body.**

49. Your pancreas weighs only 3 ounces, yet it produces 32 ounces of digestive juices each day. It is far cleverer than any machine we could invent as it quickly produces exactly the right type of digestive chemicals, at the right times, and in the right quantities for breaking down the wide variety of foods that we put into our mouths.

50. Food spends an average of 3–4 hours in the stomach, three hours in the small intestines, and 10 hours to 2 days in your 6 feet of large intestines.

51. Believe it or not, your digestive tract is also unique in that it is the only organ system that has its own brain. This "enteric nervous system" contains over 100 million nerve cells (neurons), and receives, and sends messages to your brain, gall bladder, and pancreas. These messages can range from euphoria (95% of the serotonin—a mood determiner, is stored in the gut) to nausea.

# EMBRYOLOGY

At what point in the developing embryo does he or she finally become human? Why do so many simpler forms of life resemble the primitive stages of the developing human? When does life really begin? These, and many other important questions, are way too complicated and important to be tackled here, but the amazing list of facts below is a fun glimpse into the fascinating world that you and I experienced while waiting impatiently to be born (many of us have tempered our enthusiasm since, however). The genetically coded forces that have turned the single-celled organism destined to become you into the most amazing and complex collection of cells in the universe, are both unbelievably complex and indescribably wonderful.

1. Comparing our size and lifespan with those of other animals, humans are born 2 months prematurely (which explains why we're born pink and wet, I guess—we're just not done yet). This anomaly is motivated by the continued development of our comparatively large brains.

2. Just at birth, the baby undergoes some miraculous self-surgery. A hole in the heart (Foramen Ovale), a temporary opening between the upper chambers of the heart (there because the mother has been providing oxygen until birth), is rapidly healed as millions of specialized cells rush in to fill the spot within the first year after birth.

\* In approximately 30% of us, however, a small hole persists; sometimes even into adulthood.

3. During early embryonic stages, nerve cells develop in the baby at a rate of 250,000 PER MINUTE (that's an average of 4167 cells every second!). And if this isn't impressive enough, at 5 months in the uterus, the baby accelerates nerve cell development to a rate of 200 million per minute.

\* If these neurons were people, at this rate of growth, the entire population of the world could be replenished every half hour.

4. The first taste buds develop in the fetus at only 7 weeks following conception–while bone doesn't begin developing from cartilage until 9 weeks.

5. A baby is born with over 350 "bones" (mostly cartilage), some of which immediately begin to fuse into the 206 bones which adults carry around (actually, which carry *us* around).

6. The developing embryo and fetus (the changeover in names occurs at two months of age):
   ➤ at three weeks has a heart beat independent of the mother's, and a groove that will become the nervous system;
   ➤ at four weeks has differentiated eyes, brain, spinal cord, lungs,
   ➤ stomach, and intestines;

- at five weeks is the size of a pea; the head is 1/3 of its volume;
- at six weeks has webbed fingers and toes, plus mouth, lips, tongue, and tooth buds. E.K.G. brain waves are now detectable;
- at seven weeks, the first movements are made, the baby weighs
- 1/30 of an ounce (that's about the weight of one Skittles
- candy), has swollen fingertips, and a lens in each eye;
- at eight weeks, is 1" long, and the first bones are now
- beginning to fuse, and almost all organs are in place;
- at nine weeks, the head is ½ of the baby's length, and now has foot and finger prints unlike those of any other person in the world;
- at 14 weeks, the head and body are now in proportion, and for the first time, the legs are longer than the arms. The baby swallows; there may be secretions into the amniotic fluid; thumb sucking begins (a good indication whether he or she will eventually be right- or left-handed), and the fingernails begin to grow;
- at 16 weeks is about 6" long, weighs 7 ounces (about the weight of a can of tuna fish), and completely fills the womb:
- at 20 weeks shows a few spoons-full of blood pumping around the body. The baby weighs ½ pound, is covered with fine, protective hair (lanugo), and is complete with eyebrows and eyelashes;
- at 24 weeks it is evident that the baby can now hear sounds from the internal environment, and at 32 weeks responds to music and voices from outside.
- During the last 8 weeks of development, little physical change is apparent, but now the brain and senses develop rapidly.

7. The average weight gain for the expectant U.S. mother is 29.2 pounds (I haven't been able to find any statistics on the fathers).

8. Less than 5% (one in 20) of newborns arrive on the expected due-date (and I don't just mean 9 months after the expected marriage date).

9. During fetal heart development, the human heart passes through several stages resembling the hearts of animals farther down on the development scale. For instance, at first, as a single-chambered heart, it resembles that of a fish. When it divides into two chambers, it resembles that of a frog-like amphibian. In its three-chamber phase, it resembles the heart of a reptile (like a snake). And finally, when it becomes a four-chambered heart, it is mammalian—a most efficient design, which allows us to call ourselves "warm blooded".

10. Every one of us spent about ½ an hour of our lives as a single, fertilized cell (ah, those were the carefree times).

11. Have you ever wondered why males have nipples at all? It's because during the developmental stages in the womb, up until about 6 weeks of age, we were all female in design. Only after that point did about half of us develop some of the characteristics that would eventually make us male (temporarily internal testicles, longer vocal cords, a love of tools, etc.).

* The amazing thing is that at this same 6 weeks, you were just about the size of a pea.

12. An average of one in 32 children is born with some sort of birth defect (not yours or mine of course). Most of these are non-life threatening (ex: cleft palates, external tails, webbed digits, etc.). In most cases, the defect is fixed immediately, and the "owners" never find out they were born less than perfect.

13. Many garden plants have more DNA (deoxyriboneucleic acid-genetic information) in each of their cells than we do in ours.

14. A newborn baby is a magnificent organization of 2.6 trillion cells.

* If these cells were as large as BBs, that would be enough to fill an acre of land to a depth of 119 feet.

15. 98% of babies are born with blue eyes. The color changes from a few minutes to a few days later, if it is genetically destined to do so

(I imagine this has caused more than a few tense moments between new, brown-eyed parents)

16. The bones that compose a newborn's skull aren't as rigidly attached together as yours are. Fibrous connective tissue joining the newborn's bones (fontanelles) allows the head to mold itself as necessary during the delivery process, and for the rapid growth of the brain.

17. 258 new babies are born into this world every minute. That's an average of 4 new earth residents every second. On the average, fellow human beings die at a rate of 1.8 per second.

18. One out of every 2000 babies is born with a visible tooth.

* Some primitive societies in the world today will kill babies born with a visible tooth, fearing that this event is a bad omen for the tribe.

19. For the first 6 weeks, babies cry without releasing any tears (unfortunately, the same can't be said for their overworked mother—or even dad, when the hospital bills arrive).

20. Women who are pregnant shouldn't change cat boxes because of certain transmissible diseases carried by cats (see "zoonosis" and *toxoplasma Gondii*).

21. Interestingly, babies born during the month of May are reported to weigh an average of 200 grams more than those born in any other month (200 grams is about the weight of a VHS tape).

22. A baby's body is composed of 75% water, while an adult's is about 65% water (which may explain all the drooling).

23. If all of the DNA in your body (see #13) were joined together and then stretched out, the strand would reach to the moon and back 3000 times, and yet all of it could be put into a box the size of an ice cube! In one type of body cell, the DNA strand can reach 10 feet in

**length, yet is only 80 *billionths* of an inch wide (and invisible except under the lens of a powerful microscope).**

\* That relationship is equivalent to a typical string (1/25th inch wide) stretching 242 times *around the world.*

**24. DNA replication during cell division is so precise that its accuracy is equivalent to an error of less than *one letter* in an entire set of the *Encyclopedia Britannica*, yet from these few errors come our mutations.**

**25. At the end of the first month of development within the uterus, the fetus is already 10,000 times the size it was as a fertilized egg.**

\* That's equivalent to growing from the size of a softball to the volume of a two-car garage...in one month; or you growing to about one third the size of the Washington Monument.

**26. Studies show that newborns see the world upside down because it takes time for the brain to adjust to "righting" the inverted image sent from each eye (although a complete understanding of how the brain processes information makes this concept fairly moot).**

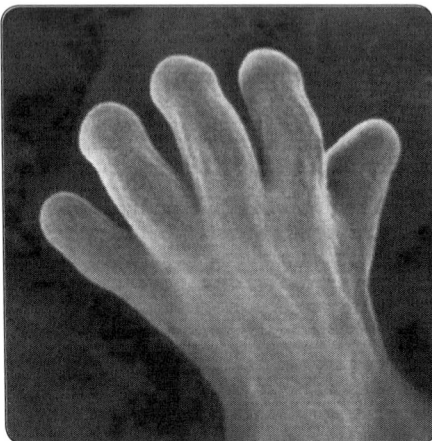

**27. A fetus's hand starts out looking like a paddle. Fingers form as non-finger-like cells around the "finished product" are reabsorbed by the body—sort of like a sculptor chiseling a statue from a slab of granite.**

**28. More babies are born between 3 & 4 a.m. than during any other time of day.**

29. On average, male babies spend one day less in the womb, but weigh one ounce more than a female baby at birth. Nobody seems to have an explanation (or perhaps care) why.

30. Medical professionals disagree as to why new mothers suffer through morning sickness. One theory is that this is one way to protect the embryo from subtle toxins the mother might be ingesting.

31. On average, babies crawl 60 miles on their knees (which generally have no knee caps), before they rise to walk

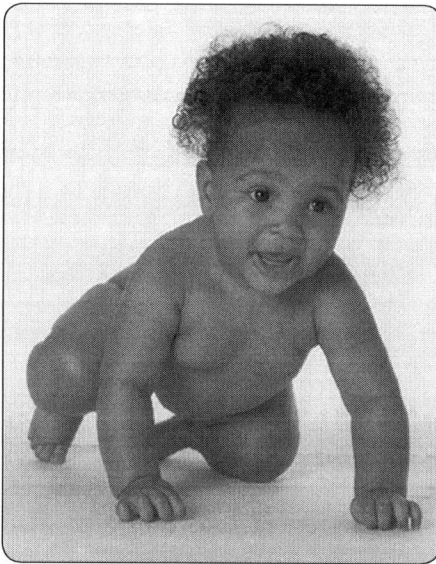

32. Until about 6 months, a baby gently submerged under water won't breathe (diver's reflex). Any water going into the mouth during the experience is shunted into the stomach.

# The CIRCULATORY SYSTEM

Much like the super highways and byways that criss-cross the inhabited wold, including each and every city street, dirt road, and driveway we depend on to move important things from place to place, our amazing circulatory system is in charge of transporting "goods" to, and by-products from, almost every cell in the body. It's pretty obvious that a sudden closure of the roads in our country would mean a quick cut-off of supplies, economic strangulation, and for all but the most prepared of us, our rapid demise. In a similar manner, the breakdown of the body's circulatory system means starvation and a quick death for each of our body's 70 trillion cells. Blood delivers vitamins, minerals, and other essential nutrients from digested food. It also carries hormones from the specialized glands which regulate our body functions. It delivers "troops" to fight infections and provides for the cleansing of each cell by exchanging carbon dioxide for oxygen, and removing other wastes via the kidneys. Statistically, when we humans eventually die, it is usually due to a breakdown in this remarkable system.

**1. During your lifetime (the average American lives 28,000 days), you make more than 10,000 *pounds* of red blood cells (erythrocytes) in the marrow of the long bones of your body, as well as in your ribs, skull, and back bones (vertebrae).**

\* 10,000 pounds is about the same weight as a typical African elephant (*Loxodonta Africana*) or 6 Volkswagen "Beetles."

---

**2. Your body *replaces* about 200 BILLION of these red blood cells *every day* (about 120,000,000 per minute). However, each one of them lives out its lifespan in an average of 4 months.**

\* That's about 2 million red blood cells produced each and every second; which is about the same number of M&Ms it takes to fill a typical bathtub to overflowing—or the number of people living in Chicago—*each second!*

---

**3. Each erythrocyte travels through the circulatory system an average of 75,000 times before it returns to the bone marrow to die.**

\* That's an average of 625 times through the body each day it lives—supplying nutrients to each one of 70 trillion customers, the cells.

---

**4. The clotting mechanism (constantly repairing small "bleeders" in your body) is so fast and efficient that if all of the blood in your body were to begin clotting at once, you would essentially solidify in 20 seconds.**

**5. By age 70, your heart will have beat an average of 2.5 *billion* times, and will have rested (between beats) a total of 40 years.**

\* How many is 2.5 billion? If one *drop* of water dripped for every heartbeat, enough water would have fallen to fill the average backyard swimming pool.

---

\* If beats were BBs, that would be enough to completely fill two public transit buses!

---

\* If heartbeats were whirring hummingbird wings, 2.5 billion beats would equal the number of "flaps" made by the little guy *if* you could keep him in the air for

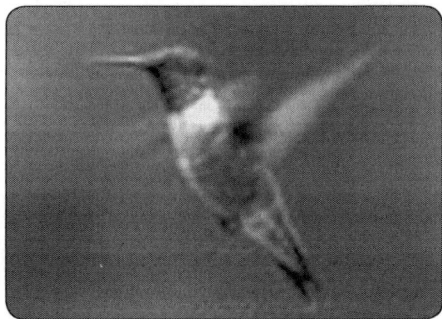

about a year and a half (By the way, a hummingbird expends so mush energy just flying, that if a 170 pound man were to do likewise…for only one day…he would expend so much energy he would have to eat 280 pounds of hamburger, or twice his weight in potatoes to not lose body-weight…and in the process, he would excrete over 100 pounds of sweat) .

**6. The human body contains approximately 62,000 miles of blood vessels— enough to reach around the world 2½ times.**

**7. Your 10 ounce heart beats an average of 100,000 times every day (many more if you are running a marathon, or are in love).**

* If you *could* squeeze a tennis ball at this same rate, for a day; at the end of that day, you would have generated enough total force to lift a small car about 5 feet into the air (and yet your heart does all of this work, stimulated by electrical impulses of only 1/25 of a volt).

*During the average night's sleep, your heart expends energy equivalent to carrying a 30-pound pack to the top of the Empire State Building.

**8. The human heart weighs only 11-14 ounces, yet at the end of the day, it will have pumped 2000 gallons of blood—over 600 pounds of the valuable fluid each hour.**

* That's enough to fill a car's gas tank every 10 minutes, or approximately 25 to 30 million gallons in a lifetime.

* It is enough blood to fill the average sized backyard swimming pool in 25 days—and enough to fill the Rose Bowl to the top in a lifetime.

**9. A three-year-olds body contains 2 pints of blood, while an adult's contains 5 times more (a little over a gallon).**

**10. At rest, the adult male heart pumps an average of 10 pints of blood per minute, while the female heart pumps eight (one gallon). During stress, your heart can pump as much as 5 *gallons* of blood every minute.**

**11. Each cubic millimeter of a man's blood (about 1/40 of a *drop*) contains 4.6-6.2 *million* red blood cells, while that of a woman's contains 4.2 to 5.4 million.**

\* If each red blood cell (erythrocyte) were the size of a marble, 5.4 million of them (remember—that's the number of red blood cells in only 1/40 of a drop) would fill an ambulance to the roof.

**12. When your heart beats, it creates enough pressure to squirt blood 30 feet (Reference: Halloween II—just kidding).**

**13. Without any assistance, a 3 mm wound will usually stop bleeding on its own within a minute. Amazingly, the chemistry that keeps blood flowing in the body, and the chemistry that clots it and allows wounds to heal, are both made in the liver.**

**14. It takes about 170 heart beats (an average of 1½ minutes) for a newborn's heart to reach optimum output.**

**15. Sniffing crayons actually lowers blood pressure. It's called the Andrews-McMeel Response. Explanation? Nobody knows for sure. My theory is that the smell of crayons simply helps us recall less hectic days.**

**16. Adults have approximately 30 *trillion* red blood cells in their bodies.**

\* 30 Trillion M&Ms would fill the Houston Astrodome three quarters to the top.

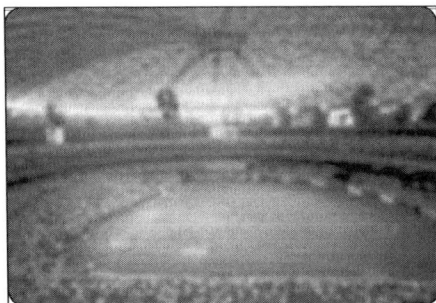

**17. Small as red blood cells are (if you lined up 500 of them, they would only measure 1/50 of an inch, or the width of a sewing needle, across), they are so numerous that if you were to lay**

yours end to end, they would reach halfway to the moon (which is about 230,000 miles away).

18. Despite the huge numbers of red blood cells contained in the human body, over ½ of your blood (55%) is actually a clear liquid called plasma.

19. Unlike the electrical system for the rest of your body, bundles of heart tissue fibers generate their own electrical current. If cut from the heart, cardiac tissue will beat independently, with no signal from the brain.

20. The electrical current generated within the heart is equivalent to only one *millionth* of the current running through a 100 watt light bulb, yet this tiny current produces the strongest muscular contraction in the body. Electrically, the heart is so extremely efficient that it converts over 50% of the fuel it uses (glucose) to energy. The most efficient automobile converts only 25% of its.

21. Blood accounts for about 1/16 of your body weight. If you weigh 150 pounds, nine pounds of you is blood—a little less than the weight of your head.

22. In addition to the erythrocytes and plasma, the blood also contains 7,000-50,000 white blood cells (leukocytes) *per drop*, depending on your body's need to fight off pathogens (germs) at the time. These are produced in the bone's marrow at an average rate of 7 million per minute.

23. If all of the blood vessels in your body were opened up and spread out, their surface area would cover 6-7,000 square meters—the area of a football field (and then you'd die of course).

24. The total surface area of all of the red blood cells (erythrocytes) in your body would cover 3-4,000 square meters. That's about 2000 times more than the area covered by your skin.

**25.** If you gain one pound of extra body fat, your heart has to work hard enough to circulate blood through an estimated 200 *miles* of added blood vessels. It's going to take more effort from the heart to do this, and that's one of the reasons why your blood pressure goes up as you gain weight.

**26.** The natives who live high in the Andes Mountains (where the air is thin) can have more than two extra quarts of blood in their bodies. Modern marathon runners have occasionally taken advantage of that biological adaptation by sleeping in sealed bedrooms with the air pressure and oxygen content adjusted to that of high altitude locations.

**27.** All of the blood in your body flows through your lungs for re-oxygenation an average of once every minute.

**28.** A single red blood cell can leave the heart, travel to the big toe (where it unloads its nutrients and oxygen and picks up the by-products of cellular respiration), and return to the heart in as little as 20 seconds

*1/3 of a mile per hour might not seem too speedy, but to put it in perspective; compare our size to that of a red blood cell and it seems as though it is traveling through the body at a speed of about 1,400 miles per hour).

**29.** Blood is supplied abundantly to every part of the body *except* for the fingernails, cartilage, some parts of the eye, and the inner ear (where the sound of your own pulse would be deafening).

**30.** The largest blood vessel in your body (the aorta) comes directly out of the heart and is about the diameter of a garden hose. It would take 160,000 capillaries (the smallest blood vessels), to fill up the lumen (inside cavity) of your aorta.

**31.** Almost none of the more than 50-70 *trillion* cells in your body are more than 1/2000 of an inch (50 microns) away from a thin-walled capillary (which supplies it with oxygen and nutrients).

32. Each of the capillaries in your body is so small that the blood cells pass through them in single file. Fifty capillaries, laid side to side, would only be as thick as a single strand of your hair.

33. Capillaries are so small and numerous that if you were to accidentally slice off a piece of your finger the size of a pea, you would have sliced through about 60,000 of them.

* If they were as thick as straws (as are many of your larger vessels), 60,000 of them would equal a bundle the size of a semi-truck.

34. Capillary walls are so thin that body water and other fluids flow continually in and out through them. Although each capillary leaks only a small amount, there are so many of them that the combined flow in and out of the cells of your body amounts to about 62 *gallons* of fluid each minute.

35. The only muscle in the body that exerts comparable contractile force to the heart muscle is the woman's uterus during the birth of a baby (however, Mom doesn't have to keep up this uterine workload 24 hours a day, for an entire lifetime—thank goodness).

36. One effect of a person's heart rate slowing down during sleep (believe me, it does) is that a large percentage of the body's capillaries become inactive.

37. Although your heart represents only about 1/200th of your body weight, it requires 1/20 of your blood supply and 1/10 of your body's oxygen supply (that's 10 times the nourishment required by any other body organ).

38. The circulatory system acts as both a delivery boy (oxygen and nutrients to the 60-70 trillion customer cells) and garbage man (waste products from the cells, to the lungs and kidneys).

* By the way; 60 *trillion* "customers" (body cells) is equal to 10,000 times the number of humans on the earth, about 600 times the number of bacteria living

on the surface of your body as we speak (OK, read), or enough BBs to completely fill the Empire State building 3 1/3 times.

**39. In the time it takes you to blink your eyes, 1.2 million erythrocytes have reached the end of their 120-day life span and perished.**

* How many is 1.2 million? If you tried to count all of the red blood cells that died during your eye-blink, and did so at one per second, it would take you 14 days to complete the task (and during *that* excitement-filled time you would have lost and replaced 2,904,000,000,000 more).

**40. Fully 15% of young women have been diagnosed with a condition in which one of the valves in the heart (bicuspid, or mitral) is slightly prolapsed. This means that a little blood ends up going the wrong way every time the heart beats (see: murmur).**

**41. Your heart beat 100,000 times yesterday, and during that time, your bone marrow produced 175 *billion* replacement red blood cells (no wonder you're tired).**

* By the way; If you decided to count to only *one* billion (at one per second), it would take you 31¾ years to finish.

**42. The liquid inside young coconuts can be, and has been, used as a substitute for blood plasma (however, even in a pinch, the Red Cross refuses to collect from generous coconut trees).**

**43. The inner layer of the arteries (Tunica intima) produces a gas (nitric oxide) which actually keeps the vessel open for optimum blood flow. When diseases (some hereditary, some caused by smoking, etc.) damage this inner layer, blood flow to the lungs and rest of the body is decreased.**

**44. An adult human in decent physical condition might have an average heart (pulse) rate of about 60 beats per minute, while that of a human in less than decent shape can average about 80 beats per minute. That difference amounts to an additional 30,000 beats every day...or 550 million additional beats *if* you survive to age 70.**

45. Emotional stress can play a huge part in triggering heart attacks. During the 30 days following September 11, 2001, throughout Washington and New York, heart attacks (Myocardial Infarctions) increased *threefold* compared to happier days before that awful event.

# THE INTEGUMENTARY SYSTEM

Were you aware that in addition to "keeping your insides in," your skin is continually performing a long list of absolutely critical chores for you? Here's just a quick summary of some of the reasons you are really, really glad you are covered with it (check below for some fun details). To begin with, poke holes in it; the outside world gets in, you get infections and may even die. If you find yourself suddenly stripped of your skin during a good rainstorm, folklore has it that you would drown (but face it, at this point, would water really be your main concern?). Without a properly functioning layer of integument wrapped around us, we would quickly become either too hot, or way too cold, supersensitive or insensitive to pain and pressure, infected, dehydrated, flaky, and bald. Not only that, we would have a very hard time telling one person from another, because race, face, and gender are, to a large extent, communicated by each and every one of our amazing suits of skin.

**1.** During his or her lifetime, the average human will grow a total of 500 miles of hair on their body (gender really doesn't make much of a statistical difference).

**2.** Humans shed about 600,000 particles of skin (clumps of skin cells) *every day*. That's about 1.3 pounds (about the weight of a cheap loaf of bread) per year, for a total of approximately 88 pounds (40 Kg) over a lifetime (about ½ of my weight).

* That's enough shed skin to fill 17½ of the 5-pound bags of flour, or 2 of the really big bags of dog food.

* We actually shed more skin than a snake—just not all at once.

**3.** About 60-70% of the dust in the average house is composed of human skin (if you have pets, the percentages can shift a bit; see "dander").

**4.** On average, humans will shed and re-grow their dead, outer layer of skin (epidermis) every 27 days.

**5.** In all, we grow about 100 completely new suits of skin (all three layers), during our lifetime (I don't know about you, but my suit has been coming back a bit wrinkled lately).

**6.** The total skin covering that you wear (minus subcutaneous fat) weighs about 6-10 pounds, making it the heaviest organ of the body (although some anatomists consider skin an "organ system" because of its complexity).

**7.** Each square inch of skin can have 32 million bacteria growing on it (obviously, more in some locations than others).

* On your entire body, that *could* amount to 16 *times*—in bacteria—the number of humans living on planet Earth (most of whom would probably avoid you like the plague).

**8. OK now take a close look at the back of your hand—each square** *inch* **of skin there contains:**

- ➤ **20 feet of blood vessels**
- ➤ **19 million cells**
- ➤ **45 large hairs**
- ➤ **90 oil (sebaceous) glands**
- ➤ **100-650 sweat glands**
- ➤ **9,000 sensory cells, including**
- ➤ **600 pain receptors, 134 yards of nerves (for a total of 45** *miles* **in the entire skin layer)**
- ➤ **36 heat sensors, and**
- ➤ **750 pressure sensors (17,000 per hand) ...and yet in some areas, it can be as thin as ½ the thickness of this piece of paper.**

**9. The skin of a typical adult female can cover 17 square feet of body, while that of the typical male covers over 20 square feet (about 3600 square inches).**

\* That's about the same surface area as the "skin" of a Volkswagen.

**10. Like fingerprints, each human has a unique set of tongue prints (but it's much harder to get the ink off afterwards).**

\* By the way, identical twins have almost identical everything *except* finger-prints. It seems that DNA does not determine finger skin patterns.

**11. Fingernails grow almost four times faster than toenails do; and longer fingers grow them the fastest. Over the course of one year, fingernails grow an average of one inch. They take about 6 months to grow from base to tip. In a lifetime, we grow approximately 100 feet of finger and toenails (about the length of three school busses).**

**12. There is an average of 55 hairs in each one of your eyebrows (That's 110 for both of course... and a bunch more for those of you with uni-brows). An eyelash lives an average of 150 days before it falls out. During a lifetime, the total length of the eyelashes we shed amounts to about 95 feet. Eyebrow hairs last an average of 3-5 months while scalp hairs typically last about 5½ years.**

**13. The thickness of your skin varies from ½ mm on your eyelids (less than the thickness of this piece of paper) to more than 5 mm on your palms and feet.**

**14. The typical human has between 90,000 and 140,000 hairs on his/her head. Blondes average 140,000; brunettes, 110,000; and red-heads, 90,000.**

* It should be noted that I myself pull the statistical average down a few hairs.

**15. If you happen to be an adult Caucasian, your body is presently growing an estimated 4-5 *million* hairs.**

* How many is 5 million?:

a.   the number of pancakes in a stack 20 miles high,

b.   the number of dollar bills in a stack 200 feet *higher* than the Empire State Building,

c.   about the same as the number of hot dogs consumed in the United States every *two* hours,

d.   the number of gallons of milk consumed *every four* hours, and

e. the number of *pounds* of potato chips consumed during last year's Super Bowl.

**16. Comparing numbers of hairs only, you are actually as hairy as a gorilla. Only your body hairs are finer (hopefully).**

* By the way; as hairy as you are, some species of spiders have 5 times more hairs on their little bodies than you do.

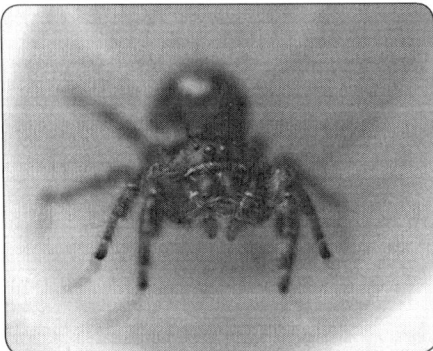

**17. The hair on your head is made of the same stuff as hooves, antlers, and claws. It is called keratin, and except for bone, will decompose much more slowly than the rest of your body when you die.**

18. If your hair is curly, it is because each individual shaft of hair is oval in cross-section instead of round, like that of your straight-haired friends.

19. The color of your hair comes from a pigment called melanin. It is the same chemical that determines (by activity level, not quantity) whether your skin will be lighter or darker. In redheads, however, the pigment is richer in iron. By the way, if you have little or no pigment left in your hair, the melanin has been replaced with *air*, and your hair is white.

* Notice how I refrained from self-deprecating and tacky references to terms like "airhead."

20. The average scalp hair grows 1/100 inch each day (3.65 inches per year). This means that the total growth of hair on the head of the average blonde is 120 feet *per day* (that's 4 school bus lengths). During a given year, average combined hair growth on the scalp alone is 8.5 *miles*, and the total growth for all of your bodily hair is a little over 12 miles.

* The average male grows and then removes 20 feet of facial hair every day.

21. Because of periodic slowing (and, for some of us, disappearing), the average growth of a single scalp hair over a lifetime is a little over 6 feet.

22. Intelligent people tend to have proportionally more zinc and copper in their hair.

* Quick, eat some oysters !

23. Fingertips are so sensitive that they can detect movement as little as one 1/1000 of a millimeter (one micron).

* Comparing a micron to the thickness of a human hair is equivalent to comparing the thickness of that hair to the thickness of a straw.

**24. A rope made from 100 human hairs is strong enough to lift a man. (However, Rapunzel's tower would still have had to be mighty short).**

**25. When you die, your hair continues to grow for a couple of months afterwards.**

**26. Over your entire body, the skin is covered with approximately 2½ million sweat (sudoriferous) glands. One type (eccrine) is primarily for cooling; the other (apocrine) is located mainly in the arm pits and groin, and essential for both cooling and the secretion of certain body wastes.**

**27. Although microscopic, the sweat glands on your body, and the tubules connecting them to the outside world, have a combined length of approximately 250 *thousand* feet (47 miles).**

**28. The average pillow (like the one on your bed right now) may contain up to a million shed-skin-eating dust mites munching happily therein.**

* The weight of your pillow actually increases as these tiny arachnids multiply, do their munching thing, and then die.

* Just to add some perspective: if you decided to count the little guys contained in the average pillow, at one per second, counting day and night, it would take you about 11.6 days to finish (and then you'd die from sleep deprivation).

**29. The average adult sweats (for cooling purposes) about 3 pints of perspiration each day, while up to 4 gallons per day can be produced by an extremely hard-working (or extremely nervous) man.**

* Just from your fingertips, you will sweat about two thimbles-full during the next 12 hours.

**30. Sweat doesn't smell! It is actually sterile (like urine) until it reaches the outside. There, it acquires its odor from contact with the fecal material of bacteria that are abundant in certain smelly areas.**

31. On your body, groups of touch sensors lie closest together in your fingertips (about 1/10 of an inch apart, which, by the way, is the reason why the raised dots in Braille letters are about 1/10 inch apart).

32. Your eyebrows form natural sweat bands over your eyes, while eyelashes (and ear hairs) keep bugs out (this is all well and good, but the BIG mystery is why these hairs continue to flourish on my face, while scalp hairs continue to diminish—now there's a question).

33. Even if you are 90 years old, your visible skin is only about three *weeks* old. So why does yours appear slightly older each year? One reason is that underlying structural support (collagen and elastin) has been breaking down...mostly from the cumulative effects of smoking and/or U.V. rays from the sun (or tanning booths).

34. We grow a total of over 7 feet of nose hairs during our lives (mostly, I noticed, when other hair growth seems to be slowing down...sort of an ironic compensatory effect, you'll have to agree).

35. During his lifetime, the average male spends a solid 145 days shaving (over 20,000 times).

36. Hairs grow, and then seem to rest for a period. At any given moment, 90% of our hairs are growing, and 10% of them are resting.

37. The eyelid is covered with the thinnest skin on the body.

38. The average human loses about 100 hairs from his/her head every day. That amounts to almost 36,500 hairs per year; about 1/3 of the total on the average head (it's a good thing that, for the lucky ones, replacements are constantly filling in).

39. The fastest growing (non-injured) tissue in the body is bone marrow. The next fastest is hair.

40. People with darker skin will wrinkle less than fair-skinned people (all other factors being the same). This is probably because of a larger quantity of active melanin, which offers additional protection against damaging U.V. rays from the sun.

41. In the United States, one in 19 people is adorned with naturally occurring red hair.

42. The collagen strands which give skin strength and structure, are stronger than steel wires of the same size, and yet are destroyed by U.V. radiation from the sun or tanning beds.

43. Skin grafts (for burns, etc.) are usually grown from the circumcised foreskins of babies. The cells from one prepuce can be cultured in a lab to the size of a tennis court.

44. The working male can easily sweat enough during a hard day at work to fill a six-pack (however, this is *not* to suggest justification for re-hydration from similar containers).

45. Beards are the fastest growing hairs on the human body. They would grow to a length of 30 feet if left uncut during an average lifetime (presumably that of the male of the species).

46. If the 100,000 scalp hairs of a "follicularly-blessed" person were woven into a rope, it could support the weight of 12 *tons* !

\* –about the weight of 3 average size elephants (Elephas Indicus), or 240 female gymnasts.

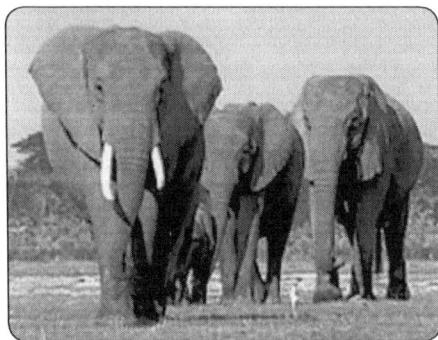

47. In case you were wondering, a "hairbreadth" is officially defined as 1/48 of an inch.

48. The outer layer of dead skin is composed of six-sided cells (sometimes called "squames").

With just the ordinary wear and tear of washing, dressing, and moving around, we rub off a half a million squames every day, which are replaced as new epidermal (that dead outer layer we are talking about) cells file forward to take their place.

49. Skin pigment (melanin) is so concentrated and intense that the difference in the amount of activated pigment between a black and white person's body wouldn't even fill a thimble.

50. Some scientists think that the tears from a crying person are different from "normal" tears in that "crying" tears contain increased amounts of the same chemicals that make you feel sad in the first place (certain neurotransmitters). Your sadness actually flows down your cheeks (and eventually, hopefully, you begin to feel better).

51. In most women, the left breast is slightly larger than the right (the breast is included in this section because it is, in reality, a modified sweat gland...although admittedly much more complex and wonderful).

52. Each breast has 17 independent milk producing units (lactiferous glands) which connect to the 17 ducts that lead to the nipple (papilla).

53. In a newborn infant (of either sex), hormones from the mother stimulate its breasts to produce a few drops of milk (called "witch's milk" by some—apparently even in cute babies).

54. Babies typically lose weight shortly after birth because the "milk" produced for the first four days after delivery (colostrum) contains little fat. Its immediate purpose is to clear mucus and other debris from the baby's digestive tract. It is also rich in antibodies, which protect the baby from many diseases.

55. In the soon-to-nurse female breast, newly developing fat-secreting glands (Montgomery's glands) develop in the areola (the dark area

surrounding the nipple), which will protect it from drying out and cracking during breast feeding. They also cause the areola to thicken and harden.

* Engorged breasts, cracking and drying nipples, as well as the occasional precocious baby tooth, may give an alternative meaning to the term "terrible twos"—sorry.

56. Crying is not for astronauts. In space tears don't flow, because of the lack of gravity (weightlessness).

57. The same gene that makes a person into a natural redhead also seems to help that fortunate individual cope with pain better—and perhaps even feel less pain than the rest of us.

58. Skin hairs stand on end when you get cold (or scared) because of the flexing of tiny muscles (arrector pili) which lie close to each hair. These elevated hairs trap warm air lying next to the surface, much as filaments in sleeping bags are fluffed up to trap warm air during a cold camp-out.

59. A common condition (hyperhydrosis), which affects 25% of Asians, causes excessive sweating in the extremities (hands, feet, etc.) and is almost certainly one reason why some cultures bow instead of shaking hands.

61. Each human replaces approximately 70 *million* skin cells every day. A sunburn (or suntan, for that matter) *greatly* increases this number (especially if you burn and peel). So? With every "batch" of cell replications comes a tiny percentage of mutant ones. Most die, but a small percentage of these are destined to become the very skin cancers that are growing and killing Americans at a geometrically increasing rate (especially as the atmosphere's protective ozone layer thins).

62. One source of skin needed for elbow transplants is the skin from the scrotum of cadavers (it's apparently hard to find living volunteers).

63. After we die, skin cells continue to divide for about 24 hours.

64. While most of the cells in your body are continually replaced, those in your heart, your brain, and in the lenses of your eyes are the same ones you were born with.

# SPECIAL SENSES

Your amazing senses of seeing, hearing, smelling, tasting, touching, and balance provide our brains with information about the physical world around us. The environment is analyzed and responded to more or less appropriately through complex exchanges between our wonderful senses, our nervous system, and then the other systems of the body. It is a marvel that all the information that reaches the brain (and spinal cord) is transformed from light waves, sound waves, particles, and pressure (detected by our senses in the first place) into electrical impulses, produced by those same senses. These impulses are analyzed by the brain and spinal cord, and then reacted to (a hastily moved finger, the blink of an eye, a slight shift in balance, etc.) usually within a fraction of a second. Our amazing senses bring the world to our brain, and because our instruments are so supremely accurate, we tend to not only survive by reacting properly to the environment inside and surrounding us, but to thoroughly enjoy the experience as well.

1. As you read this sentence, your eyes swing back and forth in tiny arcs at the rate of 100 times every second.

2. Wearing earphones can provide an environment that allows the growth of bacteria in your ears to increase 700 *times* within the first hour.

3. In general, women can hear slightly better than men, while men can read smaller print than women.

4. One man in 30 is color-blind, a condition inherited from his mother.

5. The average life-span of the human taste bud is 10-12 days (before it is replaced). However, replacement slows dramatically after age 70. In fact, by that age, most of us have lost about 50% of our ability to taste, and 40% of our ability to distinguish smells.

\* This is just one of the reasons why the elderly tend to grow thinner as they age.

6. It takes the coordinated interaction of over 70 different throat, face, and tongue muscles to produce human speech (and they usually perform quite well together, that is unless you try to repeat a name like "Peggy Babcock" three times quickly).

7. If you go blind in one eye, you will only lose about 1/5 of your effective vision (assuming both eyes had equal acuity to begin with). However, you will lose 100% of your depth perception.

8. Humans hear in the range of 20 Hz to 20,000 Hz (Hz=cycles or vibrations of sound waves per second). Rats hear in the range of 1000 to 50,000 Hz, dogs from 60 Hz to 70,000 Hz, bats up to 100,000 Hz, and elephants (and whales) can hear and transmit "infrasonic" sounds down to 2 or 3 Hz.

9. The total number of taste buds on the average human tongue is approximately 10,000. However, the actual number varies widely.

**Some people have as many as 500 taste buds per square centimeter, while others have as few as 5. (Does this mean that each one of us tastes food a bit differently—and how would you test for that?)**

\* If taste buds were the size of M&Ms, they would just cover your tongue—*If it were the size of a diving board.*

\* P.S. The winner for the largest number of taste buds in the animal kingdom is the catfish (!), with 27,000 on its fishy little tongue.

**10. There are taste buds located on other surfaces of the mouth *besides* the tongue. About 10% are located on the palate (roof of the mouth) and in the cheeks.**

**11. Located in the upper sinuses, the total number of olfactory (smell) receptors is about 40 million. These receptors transfer the molecular structure of the smell just inhaled into an electrical signal which the brain reinterprets as smell for you.**

\* If these receptors were the size of postage stamps, there would be enough to completely cover a football field. The total area that these olfactory receptors occupy in your nasal passage is *indeed* about the size of a single postage stamp

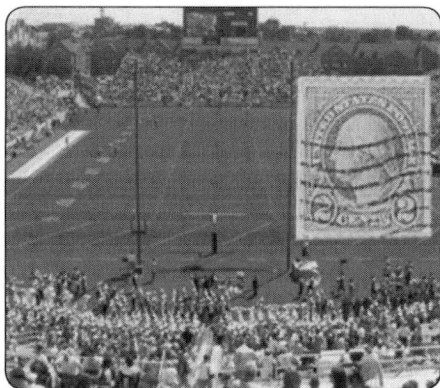

\* A dog's receptor surface area can be over 30 times larger than yours, may occupy an area the size of a handkerchief, and contain over a *billion* receptors.

**12. During waking hours, you blink your eyes between 12,000 and 19,000 times each day. That's a total of about 20 minutes per day spent with your eyes closed.**

\* By the way; that adds up to about 4 to 7 million blinks every year, or 500 million blinks during the average lifetime, for a total of 185 days per lifetime (not including sleep hours) spent with your eyes shut.

**13. Each one of your eyes has 110 million rods (which help you to see black and white) and 7 million cones (which help you to see colors).**

\* In both of your eyes, you have more light receptors (rods and cones) than there are males living in the United States.

**14. The rods are located around, but not in the exact center of the visual focus point (fovea). That's why you can sometimes pick out an object better at night by looking slightly to the side of it, and why pilots trained to look out for "traffic" in their vicinity are told to search "out of the sides of their eyes."**

**15. As stated above, when you smell something, you are actually analyzing molecules of that thing. The average smell weighs about 750 nanograms.**

\* A nanogram is one billionth of a gram; a gram is about 1/28 of an ounce; an ounce is 1/16 of a pound, so obviously it would take 597,333,300 sniffs of a smell to gain one pound of body weight (ignoring, of course, the caloric expenditure of sniffing in the first place). At one sniff per second, it would take you 20 years to gain that extra pound (so much for the fat cook/kitchen smells relationship theory).

**16. A bloodhound can smell 1000 times better than we humans can (except when they are wet, ha-ha). It kind of makes you wonder how they can stand greeting each other in the customary canine way, doesn't it? In case that sounds impressive (a dog's ability to smell, that is), a gypsy moth (the one with the impressive antenna rack you thought was for hearing) can detect a potential mate a block away from only a dozen molecules of her pheromones (sexual "fragrances") in the air. Some moths (Emperor) can detect a mate from up to 4 *miles* away.**

17. With increasing age most body parts slow down and stop growing. Your ears and nose however, continue to grow throughout your life.

18. Tears descend from over a dozen tubes above your eyes. If the naso-lacrimal gland in the base of your eye socket can't keep up with its job of draining excess tears into your nose (so *that's* why your nose runs when you cry), they end up flowing down your cheeks.

19. We have over 2000 cerumen (wax-making) glands in each ear. Old, dry ear wax is carried out to the opening (external auditory meatus) and falls out of each ear on a fairly regular basis (a careful examination of the floor around you….).

20. Newborns can typically see focused vision only as far as their noses, but almost from the beginning, can distinguish their mother's odor from others (the detection of which generally has a calming effect on the infant).

\* Experiments have also demonstrated that blindfolded mothers can recognize the smell of their own child's clothing in a pile of that from other children.

21. The average eye (and brain) can distinguish between 500 shades of gray alone, and can detect (it is estimated) more than 7 million subtle differences in color hue.

22. While our eyes are among the most acute in the animal kingdom, an owl can see a bit better. It can see a mouse 150 feet away, illuminated by only one candlepower of light (however, I have been assured by more than one of my female students that they could easily duplicate that feat... *while* perched on a table top).

23. The tongue detects things that are bitter at the back, sour on the sides, salty toward the front, and sweet on the tip.

24. It is estimated that we can distinguish 10,000 different tastes *besides* sweet, sour, salty, and bitter (and you can experience almost all of them at a good Chinese buffet).

**25. 92% of taste is actually smell (to prove this for yourself, just eat something while holding your nose). That's why professional wine tasters are called "noses."**

* With eyes closed and nose plugged, it is difficult to determine whether you are biting into an apple, or an onion. Try it on a friend if you dare.

**26. Our sensitivity to smells is actually 10,000 times *more* acute (sensitive) than that portion of taste which we detect with our tongues alone.**

**27. Five percent of the air we inhale travels upward to within ¼ inch of the brain—for smelling (olfactory) purposes.**

**28. The human eye can move from one point to another, and then refocus, in a little under ½ of a second.**

**29. For hearing acuity, we peak at age 10. From that point on, there is a steady decline (unless, of course, you accelerate things by playing drums in a rock band).**

**30. Tears contain a strong antibiotic (called lypozyme). That's why you seldom get eye infections.**

**31. The pupil of your eye (the hole through which light passes) comes from a word that originally meant "doll," from the tiny image reflected back when you look into the eyes of another (however, in my experience as a teacher, the word *pupil* seldom means *doll* ... just kidding).**

**32. Our taste buds are so sensitive that human beings can detect an increase in saltiness if only one gram of it is dissolved in 500 liters (132 gallons) of water.**

* That's as much as the weight of a thumbtack of salt, dissolved in a 4-foot-diameter wading pool, filled with 18 inches of water.

33. Olfactory nerves (those involved with the sense of smell) are actually an extension of the brain. But unlike most nerve cells, they continually replace themselves as they "burn out".

34. Because of the continual replacement of the sensory components of the olfactory system, we actually grow new smelling (olfactory) apparatus every 2 to 3 weeks, yet we never seem to forget smells, even from years in the past. Remember that special perfume or cologne from years ago that you suddenly re-encountered years later?

35. Are you ever amazed when you smell something that immediately brings back memories from years before? This is because the sensory apparatus (olfactory) for smell is located close to, and seems to have an especially direct connection with memory centers in the cortex of the brain.

* In rare individuals, a condition can exist in which the olfactory receptors are isolated from the cortex. In their case, every time they taste something, it is like tasting (and smelling) it for the first time. Wow! How would that change your life?

------------

36. Smoking cigarettes, alcohol, caffeine, hot/spicy foods, garlic, and onion dull the sensitivity of your taste buds. It takes about 24 hours for your body to cleanse the receptors again.

37. Your taste buds and olfactory receptors are most sensitive in the morning (yet another good reason *not* to skip a good breakfast).

38. You can't taste something with a completely dry mouth. It takes molecules of that something *in solution* to make the system work.

39. A perfumer can have a working knowledge of over 1000 distinct fragrances.

40. The first taste buds develop in the fetus at only 7 weeks of age.

**41. Most babies will breast-feed longer if the mother has eaten garlic, and less if the mother has had a beer (*part* of that I understand).**

**42. Most so-called aphrodisiacs (foods, potions, etc., that supposedly increase libido) have one thing in common: each contains a molecule almost identical to human pheromones (odors the body produces to attract the opposite sex). Some contain molecules that are only an atom or two different from human testosterone (a male sexual hormone).**

**43. A baby *in utero* (still inside the uterus) can respond to sounds too deep (2-3 Hz) to be heard by the adult human ear.**

* Whales and elephants frequently communicate at this level, however.

**44. On average, the pupils of your eyes become slightly larger when you are in love (even though in general, the eyes tend to be "half-shut," ha-ha).**

**45. The fluid (aqueous humor) inside your eyes is replenished every 4 hours. If the old fluid can't exit properly, pressure builds up, and you develop glaucoma.**

**46. We can distinguish between thousands of colors, yet we perform this amazing feat with only *three* structural variations in the cones of our eyes.**

**47. The optic nerve bundle is one *million* nerve fibers thick—but each nerve fiber is *extremely* thin.**

* If each fiber were expanded to one inch thick, the optic nerve bundle would measure a little under 1/2 mile in diameter. In fact, if it were only enlarged to the thickness of a human hair, the bundle would be wider than a school bus is long.

**48. Your eyes send two inverted images of the same scene to your brain. It picks out the slightly distinctive components of the images, reassembles them, and determines the distance to the object at the same time.**

49. The hearing and balance components of your inner ear are set in solid bone within the skull.

50. Your ears can distinguish between millions of subtle sound variations —far more than any known animal can claim.

51. Direction finding is possible because a sound reaches one ear (at the speed of sound—about 800 miles per hour) just slightly before reaching the other. Your amazing brain then analyzes and calculates the minute difference—and quickly enough to allow you to react within 1/20 second to say, the sound of a bee flying close to your ear.

52. The smallest bones in your body (ossicles of the middle ear) magnify the incoming sound up to 20 times. But the muscles which control these bones will contract suddenly if the incoming sound is dangerously loud, dampening the sound and preventing possible hearing damage.

53. The middle ear, which contains these three bones (malleus, stapes, and incus), is only about 1/3 of an inch across.

54. These tiny bones are unique in that don't grow any larger throughout your lifetime.

55. 15,000 tiny hairs in your inner ear (in the organ of Corti) detect, and then transform incoming sound waves into electrical signals, which are sent to the brain.

* To give you an idea of how many hairs each ear contains; if you decided to count to 15,000, at one per second, it would take you 4 hours to complete the task (and then you'd probably want to work on getting a life).

56. These specialized cells (hairs) move *hundreds* of times faster than any other cells in your body.

57. The smaller of these hair-like cells tend to die off as we grow older. The result is that we tend to lose the hearing of the higher pitched

sounds first (dog whistles, bat squeaks, our own children carrying on in church, etc.).

58. You have to be able to produce 40 distinct sounds to "master" the English language ("mastering," I presume, also requires at least a modicum of constructive time in school).

59. On average, girls learn to speak earlier than boys, but nobody knows why (or apparently has the nerve to suggest why).

60. By the age of two, many children learn to speak 2000 different words (a few of my students apparently peaked at that level—ha-ha).

61. A man's vocal cords are about one inch long and vibrate almost 120 times per second (during normal speech), while a woman's vibrate almost twice as fast. A baby's vocal cords measure only ¼ inch long (however, for sheer output volume, nature certainly seems to have favored the child).

* 120 times per second is almost twice as fast as a tiny humming bird flaps its wings.

62. Hearing isn't the most important job the inner-ear apparatus performs. Without the equipment for balance (in the semicircular canals), we would be so disoriented that we wouldn't even be able to get out of bed in the morning.

63. A combination of fluids, tiny hairs, and microscopic "slabs" (composed of the same material as common chalk) make us aware us of our head's location. We become dizzy on a circus ride because once we stop spinning, the fluid in the inner ear keeps sloshing around, sending signals and confusing the brain. The "slab," made of calcium carbonate, slides back and forth, apprising our brain of the head's backward and forward movement.

64. On a clear night, a human with good vision can see a candle burning 30 miles away (however, in some smoggy cities, you might be able to feel the heat from the candle before you can see it—ha ha).

65. The eyes are the most highly developed of our sense organs, and feed more information to the brain than any other. Fully ¼ of the nerves (cranial) arising within your brain are used to analyze and control eyesight, and roughly 80% of the sensory input that our brain processes comes from what you see.

66. The eyes are so sensitive that a good pair can distinguish between images only 1/1000 of an inch apart (that's about as far apart as 1/4th of the thickness of this sheet of paper).

67. The eyeball is about 2/3 the size of a ping-pong ball (but it doesn't bounce nearly as well).

* P.S. The eye of an ostrich is actually bigger than its brain.

_____

68. The iris of your eye (the colored portion) can open up 17 times wider in dim light than it does in bright light.

69. Your eyes have a total of over 2 *million* working parts (rods, cones, nerves, etc.), and can process over 36 thousand images per hour (with "translation" by the brain, of course).

70. When we hear the highest pitched sounds, the tiny "hair" cells in the cochlea of our inner ear move back and forth (vibrate) *less* than the diameter of larger *atoms*!

* These cochlear "hairs" are so small that 100,000 of them, bunched together, would just about equal the thickness of *one* of the hairs on your head.

_____

71. It takes only a few *millionths* of a second from the time a sound wave vibrates these "hair" cells until they generate electrical impulses (to be interpreted by the brain). By comparison, light absorption in the eye, takes *one thousand times* longer to generate its appropriate cellular responses.

**72. The sound of a needle falling on the surface of a table is so slight that the vibrations move your eardrum less than the width of a molecule. In this case, the amount of energy reaching your eardrum is estimated to be less than a millionth of a billionth of a watt—yet you can still hear it!**

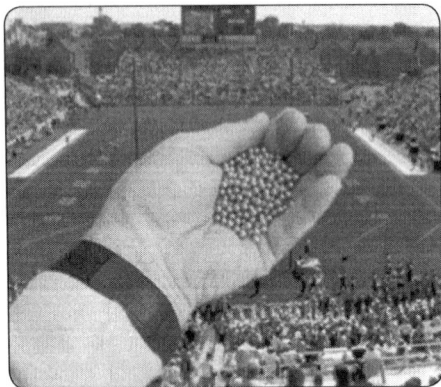

* By the way; Just to give you an idea of the size of the average molecule, each cell in your body may contain as many as 200 trillion of them. And how many is only *one* trillion? If you began to count (at one per second) to a trillion would only take you 31,500 years to complete the task. If that doesn't make things easier to grasp; one trillion BBs would be enough to fill up a football field to a depth of 35 *feet*!

**73. Tests have shown that some people (especially among the blind) can determine another person's sex (gender) solely by the smell of the pheromones (scent molecules) emanating from their body. Other tests have shown that with 95% accuracy, a blindfolded human can determine the gender of another simply by** *smelling their breath.* **Try it if you dare.**

**74. People with blue eyes are able to see slightly better in the dark than the rest of us can.**

**75. Eye color is determined to a large extent by where your ancestors came from. People who lived in sunny parts of the world generally developed dark eyes (to help block the sun's U.V. rays), while those whose ancestors lived in a world of limited sunlight had (and have) lighter eyes which let in more available light.**

**76. If the iris of your eye is heavily pigmented, it is usually brown; moderately pigmented, it is usually hazel or gray; and if slightly pig-**

mented, it reflects and scatters blue light entering (as does the sky), and they appear blue. If no pigment blocks reflected light from the retina of your eye, they appear pink, as in albinos and bad photographs.

77. You wouldn't see as clearly as you do if the exposed surface of your eyes were covered with blood vessels like the rest of your body. So this surface is unique in that it gets its oxygen supply from the tears that constantly bathe it.

78. As far as we are able to tell, only birds, man and some monkeys are able to see in "full" color. We humans are trichromatic in that we have three types of cones for color vision. Most animals have only two cone varieties (and see in blues, yellows, and grays (which explains why hunters can wear bright orange vests, and not panic the Bambies). Only the lowly rat is monochromatic, and experiences its world in shades of gray.

* Testing also seems to indicate that we humans are all color-blind at birth

79. Wearing sunglasses *without* U.V. (ultra violet A, B, and C) ray protection is actually *worse* than not wearing sunglasses at all. Why? Because they open up the eye (the pupil) and allow more damaging rays in than would enter without them.

80. When you look at a scene, there is a small, round blind spot in your field of vision (fovea), but the brain "fills it in" by supplying additional information that really wasn't there.

81. In the animal world, the cornea in the eye of the shark most closely resembles that of man's, and has even been used in surgical repair.

82. Each nostril registers smells a bit differently. Research indicates that in general, smells taken in through the right nostril seem more generally pleasant than through the left, while the left nostril detects smells more accurately than the right.

**83.** The olfactory system is so sensitive that a detected change in only *one* of the 600 chemical components of coffee can make it taste bitter to us.

**84.** Among other benefits, performing deep breathing exercises for periods of 30 minutes or more actually helps reduce pressure within the eye.

**85.** We experience pain if we are exposed to sounds over 130 decibels. (see: rock bands, pistol ranges, hungry babies, etc.)

**86.** Our ears are potentially so sensitive that a trained one can distinguish 12 *different* tones between any two keys on the piano.

* However, for some strange reason we still can't hear an echo coming from the "quack" of a duck, and nobody seems to know why.

**87.** The auditory (ear) nerve bundle is the diameter of a pencil lead, yet it has 30,000 electrical circuits within it.

* 30,000? That's about the same number of messages that a premium quality optic fiber can carry...... and the average attendance at major league baseball games last year.

**88.** The external muscles that move the eyeball around are, pound for pound, the strongest in the body (they are 100 times stronger than they need to be to do their job).

* By the way; you would have to walk (proportionately to size) 49.7 miles to get the same amount of exercise that your eye muscles get during the typical day.

**89.** The cornea (of your eye) has more sensitive nerve fibers in it than any other part of the body, and as such has a very *low* pain threshold, and is extremely sensitive to touch.

**90.** Did you know that healthy ears can actually *emit* sounds. They are very soft and seem not to be audible to the person emitting them. The sounds are thought to emanate from the central nervous system.

91. For some reason, many people who eventually develop Alzheimer's disease tend to lose their sense of smell first.

92. The human female tongue generally has more taste buds on it than the male tongue (which perhaps explains why females seem to enjoy dining out more than their male counterparts....or does it have more to do with what generally happens when the bill arrives ?—Ha ha- it's a joke!)

93. The "floaters" you can see in your field of vision are actually pieces of tissue floating around in the fluid-filled portion of your eye (vitreous fluid). They might be a distraction, but aren't medically significant, and are caused by a lifetime of wear and tear from eye rubbing, straining, trauma, etc.

94. You secrete an average of 17 gallons of tears during your lifetime (if you watch soap operas, have allergies, or a house full of teenagers, your figures may vary).

95. During the night, an ultra-thin layer of cells forms over the retina in your eye which instantly burns off as soon as light enters the room.

96. When you are sleeping, the normal position for your eyes is rolled back (up) "into your head" (known as Bell's phenomenon...no relation).

# THE MUSCULAR SYSTEM

Your muscles do much more than just move the vehicle that transports your head from place to place. A closer look should convince you that yours is one of the most efficient and well designed machines that has ever graced our planet. Your muscular system not only enables you to move, but protects vital organs, regulates heat production, as well as a dozen other essential functions.

There are actually three types of muscle tissue in your body. The ones you control are called *skeletal, voluntary, or striated* (depending on whether we are talking about their location, action, or appearance under the microscope). The second group, the ones you don't control (which run the internal functions such as digestion, breathing, gland secretion, etc.) are called *visceral, involuntary, or smooth*. The last, called *cardiac* muscle, is a very special type which makes up 90% of your magnificent heart.

1. Your muscles can generate about 40 pounds of force per square inch. If all of them pulled together at one time, you could lift about 25 *tons*, a little more than the weight of a garbage truck (and then you'd die, of course).

2. It takes 17 muscles to smile, 34 to kiss, and 43 to frown (Feeling a bit worn out lately? Take a break and smile).

3. For chewing, human jaw muscles can generate a force of 200 pounds per square inch (a crocodile can generate about 10 times that amount).

4. Inch for inch, the masseter muscle (in the jaw) is the strongest muscle in the body (the mighty tongue is reported to come in a close second).

5. The muscles surrounding your eyes (orbicularis oculus, and the extrinsic muscles) move and shut the eye (contract) an average of 100,000 times every day (about the same number of times your heart beats).

6. Human muscle cells can respond to stimuli from a nerve within 1/20 of a second (that's why your finger doesn't linger for too long on a hot stove).

7. Males lose an average of 6 1/2 pounds of muscle mass per decade after age 30, and by age 70, most humans have lost about 1/3 of their muscular strength. It isn't entirely inevitable, however. One reason for the loss is simply because we *use* them less and less as we get older (the "use it or lose it" principle).

* Less muscle mass means lowered metabolism rate, which means less efficient calorie burning, which generally means more body fat.

8. It takes the coordinated effort of over 200 muscles to merely walk across the room (if you're not well coordinated, it might even involve more).

9. The muscular system is about 25% efficient in its efforts to move bones, etc. The rest of the energy produced is expended as heat (important, but it doesn't help digging the ditch...unless it's cold outside).

* 25% efficiency, however, is almost exactly the same as that boasted by an expensive sports car.

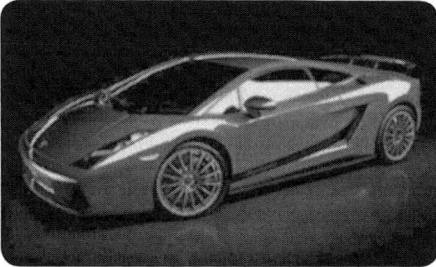

*A human body, at rest, radiates about the same amount of heat as a 100 watt light bulb.

10. The human "machine" can generate about 4½ horsepower, which is defined as the power to lift about one ton, 5 feet, in 5 seconds (amazingly, nothing is mentioned about death in the article).

11. About 50% of the average male's body weight is composed of muscle (however, bodies like Arnold Schwartzenegger used to lug around, throw the percentages off a bit).

12. We all have about the same number of muscle cells in our bodies (Arnold's are just a whole bunch longer and thicker than mine).

13. Your body has about 650 distinct muscles. That works out to an average of three per bone.

* Cats have 42 muscles in each ear (and 34 controlling just the tail).

14. Each muscle cell is thinner than a hair (a human hair is about 100 microns thick), and up to 2" long. A muscle fiber in your biceps, for example, may be only 10 microns thick and 10 centimeters long. If one centimeter is 10,000 microns long, that means that a muscle fiber may be 10,000 *times* longer than it is wide—about the same

proportions as a rope 2" in diameter, stretching the length of 5 football fields.

15. In general, our voluntary muscles come in two varieties: white (or "fast twitch"), which have limited blood supply, but which are capable of fast, but "short-winded" action (like those in the arms and hands); and the dark variety (with rich blood supply), which contract more slowly, but can perform work for much longer periods; like those in trained legs, for example.

16. It takes the interaction of 72 different muscles to produce speech.

17. With the exception of certain stages of sleep, our muscles are under a constant state of contraction. This is called muscle "tone," and is why you aren't collapsing in a heap as you read this.

18. Without salt, potassium, and calcium, your muscles can't contract (and this includes your heart).

19. The human body, magnificently resplendent as it is with its 650 muscles, has fewer of them than a caterpillar (which has about 2000).

20. The smallest muscle in the body (the stapedius) lies in the middle ear. It is a little over 1/25 of an inch long and thinner than a common thread).

21. The longest muscle in the body lies diagonally along your inner leg (sartorius) and helps you cross your legs. It is named after the "tailor," who in the old days, sat that way as he or she sewed.

22. The muscles that move your eyes are the most active muscles in your body (want to take bets as to which of yours are the least active?).

**23. When a muscle contracts, the individual muscle fibers actually contract, relax, and then contract again at about 5 times per second.**

**24. When you stand erect, your body is supported by the interaction of about 400 muscles and 1000 ligaments.**

* Most back problems arise as spinal muscles are forced to support (as abdominal muscles weaken) the average 10 pounds of "paunch" that burdens the typical male equator. The backaches that the unhappy pregnant female experiences are similarly caused, but fortunately (hopefully), this problem tends to resolve itself a few months later.

**25. A study done at the University of Minnesota indicates that people tend to stop shivering if asked to add up a list of numbers (except during a college math test, I suspect). Try it.**

**26. Humans have more facial muscles than any other creature on earth (22 on each side of the face).**

* It is said that humans communicate far more information to each other with facial expressions (part of our "body language") than we do with words.

**27. Blinking is the fastest reflex that we humans exhibit to the world.**

# The **NERVOUS SYSTEM**

S o much more than merely a complex switchboard or even the most sophisticated computer ever dreamed of, our nervous system is really who we are. OK, a bit unscientific perhaps, but understanding the true nature of this fabulous system, we end up forced to admit that in our case, the whole is definitely *far* greater than the sum of its parts. Billions of simultaneous connections may yield huge numbers of responses to a dizzying amount of stimuli—but we are humans after all. Which combination of connections causes human yearning, or ambition, or even moodiness? We just don't know. With and without our conscious awareness, and with remarkable accuracy, the nervous system continuously interprets readings from our internal and external environment and then responds to (or allows us to respond to) them. Electrically and bio-chemically driven, it is indeed the most complex collection of matter in our universe—one which we are just beginning to understand.

**1. Unconsciousness will occur about 8-10 seconds after loss of blood supply to the brain.**

**2. There are approximately 13 million nerve cells in the spinal cord.**

\* That's about the same number as dollar bills in a stack one mile high.

**3. The average human brain weighs about 3 pounds, and can consume up to 1/3 of the body's energy. It has the size and shape of an oval grapefruit, and the consistency of a bowl of Jello.**

**4. The human brain has approximately 100 billion neurons (nerve cells) which send signals to one another across 100 trillion terminals.**

\* If these neurons were stretched out, they would reach 30,000 miles (or a little over one trip around the world).

\* By comparison, the brain of an octopus (one of the aquatic world's most intelligent creatures) contains only about 300 million neurons (about 1/350th of ours).

\* 100 billion is 17 times the number of people on this planet, or almost exactly the same number of M&Ms it would take to cover a baseball field (with a 350' fence) to a depth of about 50 feet...and very close to the number of hamburgers eaten in the United States every 2 years.

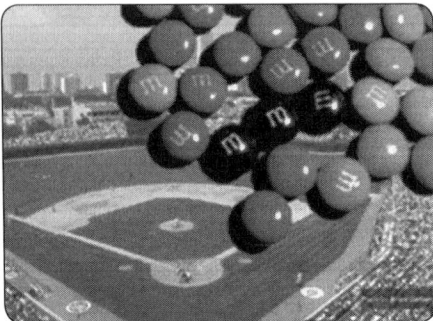

\* 100 billion is also the number of pieces of paper in a stack 500 miles high.

\* 100 trillion is approximately the number of grains of fairly coarse sand contained in a plot of beach the size of a tennis court and a foot deep—or the number of leaves on the trees of a fairly dense forest covering a million square miles (a little under 4x the area of Texas).

5. Your brain and spinal cord receive and send messages at a speed of 240 miles an hour (or 350 feet per second... about 1/4 of the speed of a .22 cal. long rifle bullet).

6. A nerve can send up to 1000 impulses every second. The transmission of impulses from one nerve to another, even at this amazing speed and rate, depends on *chemical* reactions that go on in tiny spaces (synapses) between the nerves themselves. These chemical reactions occur so rapidly that one synapse can "fire" up to 10 impulses per second.

7. The storage capacity of the average brain exceeds 4 terabytes (most home computers contain less than 3 or 4 gigabytes of memory—a terabyte is 1000 *times* a gigabyte). But this represents *just* the memory capacity, not capacity for the infinitely more complex processes of creative thinking and emotion.

8. Each neuron can connect directly with as many as 10,000 other neurons (like a really huge intersection).

* Mathematically, this actually multiplies out to more potential connections than there are *atoms* in the universe.

9. Even though the brain and spinal cord are surrounded, nourished, and protected by a little over a cup (125-150 cc) of cerebrospinal fluid. For purity requirements, a total of 400-500 cc of this amazing fluid is manufactured, used, and then replenished by the body every day.

10. Touch something hot, and the message is relayed to your spinal cord (and immediately thereafter, your brain) in less than 1/000 of a second. If you suddenly react to a hot stove for instance, it is a reflex involving just your spinal cord, arm muscles, and your poor finger. If

you suddenly feel a laudable desire to apply cold water to the area, your brain has become involved.

11. The thumb is so important to what humans do that it has a section in the brain devoted entirely to manipulating it; a section entirely separate from that of the fingers.

12. With few exceptions, your brain is larger and heavier than that of any other animal. At 40-50 ounces, it is 2-3 times the weight of any class of ape brain.

* However, while man has an average of one gram of brain material for every 44 grams of body weight, the Capuchin monkey has a ration of only one gram per only 17.5 grams of body weight. And while the weight of a whale's brain outweighs ours by 4 times, the ratio of brain to body size is only 1:8500.

* It is also interesting that, as evidenced from the size of the cranial cavity alone, cubic inch for cubic inch, the brain of the Neanderthal was bigger than yours—sorry.

13. There is little correlation between brain size and intelligence (males generally have larger brains than females). External convolutions (folds and grooves) and internal complexity explain most of the differences.

14. A baby's brain physically grows 300% during the first year of life.

15. The weight of a newborn's brain increases 1-2 milligrams *per minute*. That's up to the weight of a penny—every day.

16. A person can remain conscious 8-10 seconds after being decapitated. (What would *you* be thinking about? Eventually you'd just have to quit while you're a head. ha-ha—Sorry).

17. In the brains of musicians, there are 130% more cells in the brain's auditory section, compared to a person who is tone deaf.

18. 15% of the body's blood supply goes to the brain. Your brain consumes up to 25% of the oxygen your body takes in, yet it only accounts for about 2% of your body weight, *but* does not grow, divide, or contract like other body parts.

19. The brain also uses more energy than any other organ in the body, burning a whopping 20-33% of the body's total energy supply.

20. In each generation of human development, it is estimated that the brain has added an average of 150,000 brain cells. It is three times larger than anthropoid brains were 2½ million years ago (see #12 for one possible exception).

21. If all of the neurons (nerve cells) in the brain were to "fire" at once, it would require only enough energy to light a 10 watt light bulb (about the same size as the one that illuminates your glove box), yet the human brain generates more electrical impulses every day than all of the telephones in the world—combined.

22. One quarter of the major nerves in the brain are devoted to vision.

23. The optic nerve (to the eye) is actually an extension of the brain.

24. How healthy is your brain? Here's a test to measure the brain-body communication: Stand on one foot with your eyes closed. A "young" brain should enable you to maintain this stork-like position for 15 seconds or more (an especially good sign if you are over 40).

25. In general, the left half of your brain controls the right side of your body, and vice versa (that's why left handed people insist that they are the only ones in their right minds—ha-ha). For some reason, however, the right nostril is electrically connected to the right side of the brain, and also vice versa.

**26.** If you are right-handed, the left side of your brain deals with skills such as communication, reading, and writing, while the right side deals with artistic endeavors, imagination, etc. A left-handed person's brain usually works in the same way, but in some cases the functions of the two halves (hemispheres) are reversed.

**27.** The brain performs all of its amazing functions, fueled only by glucose, the simplest of sugars.

**28.** Nerve impulses travel across a muscle fiber in less than 1/1000 of a second.

\* At a speed of 240 mph, that impulse can travel 4 inches in your brain in approximately the same amount of time that it takes the tire of a car traveling at 60 mph to roll over a postage stamp stuck on the road.

**29.** Because of the complex way that brain tissue is folded, the outer layer (gray matter/cerebral cortex) is only a few millimeters thick, yet it accounts for 40% of the entire brain mass.

\* Definition of old age: that stage of life when you occasionally feel that you have more gray matter on the outside of your head than you have on the inside.

**30.** Mental activity helps keep the brain young. It is estimated that the brain of a college graduate who continues to learn in vocational or educational settings has a brain 2½ years "younger" than that of a high school dropout (as measured by mental acuity tests).

**31.** The pituitary gland, located deep within the brain, produces hormones (see section on the endocrine system) that govern growth, sexual development, metabolic activities (such as water balance, uterine contractions, etc.), and yet it is only the size of a pea.

**32.** The Central Nervous System (brain and spinal cord) is connected to every part of the body by 43 pairs of nerves and their branches. 12 pair emanate from the brain, and 31 pair from the spinal cord.

33. There are nearly 45 *miles* of major nerves running throughout your body.

34. 85% of the human brain is composed of water (only about 65% of the rest of the body is).

35. One small section of the brain (the thalamus) actually suppresses unimportant information. That's why, while you are reading this book, you might not notice the bird chirping outside, or even that person coming into the room. When it *is* important, however, the thalamus can make you extremely aware of an intruder, while suppressing the sound of a cat purring at your feet.

36. Over twice as many people in the United States die of Alzheimer's disease each year (approximately 100,000) as do in all of the traffic accidents combined.

37. If you had to run away from a sudden threat, a portion of the nervous system (autonomic) would immediately stop your body from digesting food and route all available blood to the "run-away" muscles in your body.

38. Size-wise, your brain stops growing at about age 15. But hopefully, intelligence doesn't (It may certainly appear slowed down in individuals wearing caps facing the wrong way, but generally we keep evolving).

39. The sending portion of a nerve cell (the axon) can be as long as the length of the spinal cord (more than 3 feet), making some nerve cells the longest cells in the human body.

\* Notice it doesn't say "largest." See Reproduction System.

---

40. Nerve impulses in the body of the elderly tend to travel more slowly than they do in the body of a youth (from 180 mph down to about 150 mph) *except* in the brain, where in most individuals, increased myelination (more of the insulating layer surrounding the

nerve) actually allows some types of impulses to travel faster as we age.

41. Past the age of 35, we lose about 10,000 brain neurons *every day* (at this rate, in another 27,400 years, I won't have any brain left at all). However, at about age 35, we also develop billions of new dendrite (nerve) connections between the nerves we *are* left with. Upon testing, short-term memory seems to decrease a bit, while long-term memory increases, compared to that of 20-year-olds.

42. A newborn baby can't detect whether a fly has landed on it or not, and almost certainly wouldn't know whether the fly was on a leg or arm. It *isn't* because there are too many nerves missing (babies have all of the billions of brain cells they need), it's because, for the present, neural pathways aren't completely organized or integrated.

43. Because of the rapid influx of new information into a baby's life, it is theorized that babies have to dream longer than adults do. According to some sleep scientists, dream-time is the period we need to sort out the experiences of the day before (so if you have no life, you should be able to get along on less sleep—right?)

44. The sound, sight, and touch of a mosquito landing on your arm may cause the firing of hundreds of thousands of neurons, but most of these signals will be "filtered out," leaving only a select few for the brain to analyze (and decide whether to have your muscles swat at it or not).

45. The human mind has an amazing ability to give meaning to images on a printed page. To show the impressive adaptability of your brain, read the following:

I cdnuolt blvelee tahy I cloud aulacity uesdnatnrd waht I was rdanieg. The phaonmneal pweor of the hmuan mnid is azmaznig. Aoccdrnig to a rscheearch sudty at Cmagrigde Uinerctisy, it deosn"t mttaer in wahy oredr the ltteers in a wrod are, the olny iprmoatnt tihng is taht the frist and lsat ltteer be in the rghit pclae. The rset can be a taotl mses and you can sitll raed it wouthit a porbelm. Tihs is bcuseae the huamn mnid deos not raed ervey lteter by istlef, but the wrod as a wlohe. Amzanig huh? (*You* might not have had much trouble with this—but it drove my spell checker crazy!)

46. The reason you can (for instance) think of eating a juicy hamburger while jumping rope is that the neural pathways for the concept of "hamburger" can continue to fire over and over, ½ of a millisecond (.0005 sec) apart, without tiring. However, some types of thinking processes *do* interfere with each other, such as talking on a cell phone while driving a car at the same time.

* As an example of this "neural synapse overlapping" try this experiment: Sit down with both feet on the floor. Now lift the right leg and swing it in a circle clockwise. With it going, lift your right arm and in the air, write the number "6". Notice how your leg changed direction? (Like the phone conversation and driving…you can't do both as well as either separately).

47. Our working memory (the very short-term memory which stores information just long enough for us to understand a concept) can hold an average of 7 digits (which is a darned good reason for telephone numbers to be 7 digits long).

48. During the first month of a baby's life, the brain synapses grow in number from 50 trillion to over 1 quadrillion (20 times more). If the baby's body weight grew as fast as its brain, it would grow from 8.5 pounds at birth, to over 170 pounds by one month old (and logistically, nursing would become a nightmare).

49. Tests done on violent male prisoners found 11-14% fewer nerve cells in the pre-frontal cortex of the brain. That's the part of the brain associated with relationships between cause and effect; action and outcome. Other studies have shown that this area of the brain often doesn't develop fully until the late teens or early 20s (which may explain the carnage encountered in the typical high school parking lot).

50. Even so, during the second half of a child's first year, this same pre-frontal cortex (also concerned with forethought and logic) forms synapses at such an astonishing rate that it consumes 2X the energy of the adult brain while doing so.

51. If the brain is surgically split down the middle (commisurotomy of the corpus callosum), an interesting thing occurs: One immediate reaction is that written words presented to the patient in the left part if his/her visual field cannot be read (alexia), and familiar objects placed in the left hand (unseen) cannot be given a name (anomia).

52. In early prenatal development, the fetus develops brain neurons at an astounding rate of 250,000 *per minute* ("huffing" dangerous chemicals can *permanently* destroy brain cells at an even faster rate than that).

53. The portion of the brain called the hypothalamus controls heart beat, body temperature, thirst, appetite, breathing rate, and functional aspects of the nervous system—and it is only the size of a cherry.

# The ENDOCRINE SYSTEM, METABOLISM and GROWTH

W hile the nervous system interprets and reacts to our internal and external environment, and responds to changes rapidly, and electrically; the endocrine system performs essentially the same job, controlling things at a slower pace, and mostly with chemicals. Glands throughout the body, which "dump" their hormones directly into the circulatory system, have a profound effect on our daily lives. These chemical "exciters" regulate daily functions including growth, reproduction, energy production, bodily fluid balance, stress reduction, and even the acidity level within each of our cells. If too much or too little of an important "thing" is happening in our body, our endocrine system detects this change from normal (homeostasis) and responds to it by releasing corrective chemistry. Although the endocrine system is often a "slow responder" compared to the nervous system, it is nevertheless pretty impressive how quickly the adrenal glands can motivate you to move when something scary jumps out at you at the spook alley.

1. Children grow faster in the springtime than at any other time of year (as do future weeds and credit card debt).

2. It is possible for an enthusiastic teenager to burn an average of 20 calories per minute while chewing gum! This would *theoretically* allow them to masticate (chew) away a pound of body weight every three hours except that (1) gum usually contains calories, and (2) gum chewing tends to make a person hungrier, due to the stimulated production of digestive juices (see Bell's rule #3: "It's never that simple").

3. The Endocrine System, systematically and precisely administers 40 different chemical hormones ("exciters") within your body.

4. Native American Indians lack an enzyme (aldehyde dehydrogenase) that processes alcohol and passes it from the body (so do 50% of Asians, and a small percentage of Blacks and Caucasians).

5. 80% of the heat escaping from your body on a cold day escapes through your head (hence the survivalists' saying that "if you want to warm your feet, put on your hat").

6. The sodium/potassium "battery" (pump) in each cell generates approximately 1/10 volt per cell. Surprisingly, that adds up to 200,000 volts per square inch!

* An electric eel, which has thousands of its cells lined up electrically, instead of being randomly scattered like ours, can produce a 600-volt lethal shock.

7. Each cell in your body produces as much electrical energy for its weight as a nuclear power plant does for its.

8. It takes 1 hour and 51 minutes of light exercise for a man in his 20s to burn 500 calories (Kcals), while it takes a woman of the same age 3 hours and 29 minutes to burn the same number. A female, sitting in a chair, takes 7 hours and 34 minutes to burn 500 calories, while a male burns calories at that same rate—while sleeping.

9. Most of your body is no more than 10 years old (I don't know about that... parts of mine certainly *look* older).

10. At puberty, most hormones are released (by the hypothalamus) during sleep, and in 90-minute bursts (which can definitely be a hair-raising experience. Sorry)

11. One of the main shocks a newborn experiences is from the comparative cold of the outside environment. It takes a full 6 months for the average baby to completely acclimatize to temperature fluctuations in the "outside world"

12. Two chemicals produced by your body control fear (adrenalin) and anger (noradrenalin). These molecules are so similar (distinguished by only *one atom*), that you can feel fear and anger at the same time (such as when your "run-away" child is found 4 hours later, hiding in the hall closet, with a big grin on his or her face).

13. The liver (deeply involved in body metabolism) is a magnificent manufacturing plant, unmatched by anything constructed by man. For the body's construction and repair needs (one of the liver's many functions) it produces 1,000,000 protein molecules *per minute* when needed.

* How many is one million, anyway? 1 million inches = 15 miles, and a million minutes = two years.

14. The liver is the body's storage battery, recycling center, health club, and "detox" unit, all in one.

15. If 80% of your liver were removed, the remainder would continue to function, and within a few months it will have rebuilt itself to its original size.

16. The hormone melatonin (produced in the tiny pineal gland in the brain) helps us sleep. Its production stops as soon as closed eyes detect light coming into the room.

**17.** We "grow" about 1/3 of an inch every night—and only at night. It starts about 1½ hours after we fall asleep. During the following day, most of that "growth" is compacted again because of the effects of gravity.

* Because of this, astronauts can temporarily grow up to two inches taller during a long space flight.

**18.** As we travel from east to west, the "jet lag" lasts twice as long as it does when we travel in the opposite direction. The main reason that jet lag is so hard on us is because hormones are produced in the body on a fairly rigid schedule, night and day.

**19.** If you multiply the height of a child on his/her second birthday by 2, it will give you a fairly close approximation of what that child's height will be as an adult. The typical two-year-old boy has grown to 49.5% of his eventual adult height, while a two-year-old girl has grown to 52.8% of hers.

**20.** Among other functions, your pituitary gland controls the growth hormones in your body. This amazing collection of highly specialized tissue is about the size of a pea and weighs a little less than a paper clip.

**21.** Located in a protected area deep in your brain, the pituitary gland has been called the body's "master gland" because it controls the chemical output of other glands in your body. The ten essential hormones it produces each day weigh a total of only 1/1,000,000 of a gram.

* That's about the same weight in hormones as *one* of the hairs on your head, cut to a section only 1/2000 of an inch long.

**22.** Compared to the chemistry of the pituitary gland, the weight of hormones released by your thyroid gland (which controls your metabolism rate—the rate at which you "burn" calories) is considerably greater. Comparatively, *its* daily output is much higher at 1/100,000 of an *ounce*. That's about the weight of 10 of your scalp hairs (that is, unless your name is Rapunzel).

23. Among other critical functions, your amazing pancreas produces insulin, which regulates sugars in the body. It is manufactured in over one million specialized cells called "islet" (of Langerhans) cells. This pancreatic production is done *in addition* to it's other job of manufacturing and releasing digestive "juices," which makes it the only combination endocrine and exocrine gland in the body. All one million of these islet cells represent only 1.5% of the 3 ounce weight of the Pancreas.

* For Islet cells, that's a total weight of 7 grams, or about the same as two unwrapped Hershey's kisses.

24. The thyroid gland regulates 1/5000 of a gram of Iodine each day. With its use, your weight, heart rate, cholesterol level in the blood, muscle strength, skin condition, eyesight, and even emotions are regulated (especially when you are angry while bent over, and squinting in disbelief at the bathroom scale, I imagine).

25. The repair of damages to, and diseases of the body, is typically accomplished during the night. These critical functions are especially accelerated between 10:00 p.m. and 2:00 a.m. (so, in general, climb into bed and heal.)

# The REPRODUCTIVE SYSTEM And GENETICS

The amazing thing about the human reproductive system (compared with that of most of the biomass on this planet) is that we are "forced" to share genetic information—the stuff that makes each one of us unique. The happy result is that during our comparatively short stay here on earth, we humans have been able to adapt remarkably well to short and long term changes in the world around us. Germs do a pretty good job of adapting too, but they have to produce a "skadillion" babies to make their system work (a scary thought for at least half of us). Not only that, but as far as we have been able to scientifically determine, simply dividing in half and creating two identical clones of ourselves, would also be far less fun. It is a remarkable thing how structural differences between the male and female reproductive systems act to select only the best genetic package from each, to be passed on to the next generation. Ours is a wonderful mixture of something most of the living world does without (pleasure), and a system that insures, with few exceptions, that the best qualities of both individuals present themselves in the next generation. Isn't it great being human?

1. Every human being (including you) spent about half an hour as a single, fertilized cell; a cell which already contained all of the information inside necessary to generate the you, you are today.

2. The mapped genome (it contains all of the genetic information supplied by our 21,000 genes) for the human body would fill 200 phone books of 500 pages each.

* If the 7 trillion nucleotides and genetic sequencing information that compose the human genome would fill say 1000 large books, the *differences* between the information describing the apes and humans would fill only 10 of those books (but vive la difference).

* Chromosomally, humans are 99.9% identical to each other, and yet no two of us are exactly alike.

3. The difference between the DNA of a human and that of an ape amounts to only 2-3% of the total. This may seem like a tiny difference, but genetically, the difference between a human's DNA and that of a mouse is only 15%.

*Genetically, we are more closely related to a chimpanzee, than a rat is to a mouse.

4. Most men have erections an average of every 1 ½ hours during sleep. However, erectile dysfunction, which affects 30 million American men (and those are the ones who had the nerve to answer "yes" on the questionnaire), may also be a negative indicator of *overall* arterial health throughout the body.

5. The largest cell in the human body is the ovum (egg), while the smallest is the spermatozoon (sperm). It takes 175,000 sperm to equal the weight of one egg. The diameter of the egg is 1/175th of an inch (slightly smaller than ¼ of the size of the period at the end of this sentence) and is the *only* human cell visible to the naked eye.

* By the way, the ostrich lays the largest animal cell in nature.

6. In the United States, the month of August averages the largest number of births—apparently there's something unusually romantic about December (or maybe it's just "cold outside").

7. The average human will have sex about 3500 times during his/her lifetime (Yes, I know that only averages out to a little under once per week, but figure in a) age of maturity, b) age of diminished activity, and c) headaches, and it all begins to make sense).

8. Human reproduction follows lunar time rather than solar (sidereal) time. Gestation is about 266 days (or 9 lunar months); the menstrual cycle is one lunar month long (28 days). Any suggestions as to why? (and does the word "lunatic" have anything to do with it?) Science wants to know.

* Incidentally; to adjust your time from solar to lunar, just subtract 2 1/3 minutes from each day.

9. The human sperm (in search of the egg) travels 1/10 of an inch per minute. It usually takes about an hour of steady swimming for the determined human sperm to reach the egg.

10. ...but considering the sperm's small size, that rate of swimming would break every free-style swimming record in the book. If the sperm were the size of its "donor," the swim to the egg would be the equivalent of swimming 10 miles (through some rather unfriendly situations and conditions, I might add).

11. A healthy human male makes from 60,000 to 120,000 sperm *per minute!* That equals 1000 to 2000 sperm *per second* (of course), for a total of up to 180 *million* sperm every day. That's enough sperm to fertilize every fecund (able to reproduce) female in the United States and Canada combined, and enough sperm produced in a month to potentially fertilize every female on the planet.

* 1000 sperm per second—that's one per millisecond; about the same speed as a housefly flapping it's wings, and the time it takes a bolt of lightning to travel from the ground to a cloud.

### 12. A typical ejaculation releases 200-250 *million* sperm.

* If each spermatozoon were the size of a drop, that would equal the number of drops in 2,500 gallons of milk (a little less than 1/2 of a milk tanker truck full.) Sperm are so small that it would take 400 of them to completely cover the period at the end of this sentence (just take my word for it).

**13.** In case you are overly impressed by human male sperm-manu-facturing capabilities, he produces about the same number of sperm as that released by a healthy hamster (puzzled? see # 18).

**14.** Three out of four human males can reach a climax (orgasm) in two minutes (however, three out of four females tend to discourage this.)

**15.** The average duration of sexual intercourse for males in the 18-24 year-old group is 12 minutes (notice the laudable implied restraint?)

**16.** A woman's sex drive (libido) is actually driven by a small amount of the "male" hormone testosterone that she has in her body (does that really surprise anybody?)

**17.** Semen contains powerful, mood-altering chemicals (testoster-one, prolactin, leuteinizing hormone, estrogen, and prostaglan-dins), which are absorbed through the walls of the vagina during intercourse, and which (in general) have the effect of *elevating moods.* (!)

**18.** Most of the material in semen is not sperm, but a fluid that pro-tects the sperm from the acidic environment of the vagina, and sup-plies nourishment for the arduous journey ahead.

19. The "life span" of the average pubic hair is 6 months. (I wonder if this figure takes non-average pubic hairs into consideration.)

20. Among other things, humans differ sexually from other animals in that:
A. Breasts are "fully" externally positioned, even when not nursing.
B. The female can enjoy sex all year long (not just when producing eggs (estrus).

21. Sex (as opposed to asexual reproduction) has allowed our species to "shuffle" the gene pool in such a way that we have been able to adapt to situations that would mean extinction for many simpler species.

22. Within 7 months of conception, the fetus has developed 7 *million* immature eggs in her immature ovary. At puberty, she has 300,000 of them left (the rest were reabsorbed by her body), of which only 300-400 will grow to maturity (less than ½ the number of sperm the male produces each second). These are released monthly (typically, first from one ovary, and then from the other) during the fecund (able to reproduce) lifetime of the typical female.

23. During the lifetime of the human male, he produces about 1½ *trillion* sperm. That's enough to populate the world 350 times over.

* If sperm were as large as BBs, 10 trillion of them would be enough to fill the typical soccer field to a depth of 240 feet!

24. Sperm can only develop at a temperature a few degrees lower than body temperature. To maintain that ideal temperature, special muscles (dartos) in the groin continually raise and lower the testicular sac (scrotum) to keep the testes the proper distance from the body. This raising and lowering effect goes on mostly unnoticed by the male, and can, by the way, be significantly influenced by tight fitting "undies".

* Elephants, whales, and bats don't have protruding scrotums; they carry their testes within their bodies (...yet another reason for their infrequent appearances on America's Funniest Videos).

**25.** It takes the human male 10 weeks to completely develop a sperm to maturity (it is an "assembly-line" sort of process).

**26.** An average of 100 *million* sperm are immediately killed as they enter the acidic environment of the vagina. Fertilization is generally a "survival of the fittest" sort of program—with an element of pure luck at the very beginning.

**27.** A mucus plug in the neck (cervix) of the uterus is 100% effective at keeping sperm out *except* for two days out of every lunar month when the plug becomes porous, and sperm are permitted entrance.

**28.** When the human female reaches orgasm, pressure within the uterus actually decreases, making passage by sperm into the uterus even easier (!).

**29.** Of the 250 million sperm that begin the journey to reach the egg, only about 100 actually do (100 out of 250 million is proportionally equal to one in 2,500,000).

\* That would be equivalent to being the winner of a Boston Marathon with 100 *times* more runners than the last one.

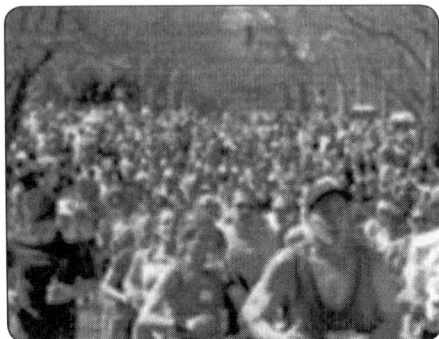

**30.** One half of all fertilized eggs *fail* to implant in the uterus and leave the body (mostly unnoticed) as spontaneous abortions.

**31.** From fertilized egg (zygote) to new-born baby, the growth rate (by weight) has been almost a *billion* times.

* That's about the same as comparing the weight of a paperclip to that of 10 blue whales (By the way: a single blue whale is so large that its *tongue* weighs more than the average elephant).

---

**32. At the beginning of the third trimester of human pregnancy (at 24 weeks), the size of the mother's heart expands so that it can pump 1/3 more blood. Her breathing becomes deeper, but her respiration rate remains the same so that her baby can get more oxygen.**

**33. In each male's testicle, there are over 350 *feet* of sperm-producing tubules (seminiferous). Each tubule is as fine as the finest silk thread.**

* 350 feet is about the length of a football field

---

**34. On their journey to the ovum, the sperm that make it to the entrance of the fallopian tubes (also known as ovarian ducts, or uterine tubes) rubs off a protective coating on its tip (acrosome), and exposes an enzyme (think "dissolving agent") which allows it (if it becomes the solitary winner) to burrow through the wall of the waiting egg.**

**35. To a spermatozoon, this barrier (the membrane of the egg) is equivalent to a wall 30 feet thick, *but* the amazing wall will temporarily soften only until one lucky sperm breaks through, and then immediately harden (as an electrical impulse travels through it), preventing entry by any other sperm.**

**36. Identical twins occur once in every 300 pregnancies. They occur when a fertilized egg (zygote) divides into two separate halves early in the dividing process. Each half then continues to develop. Fraternal twins, on the other hand, result when two (or more) eggs are released and fertilized by separate sperm.**

* In the United States, 150 identical twins are *married* to other identical twins.

---

**37. Statistically, the odds against giving birth to twins are one in 85 births; for triplets, one in 7,000 births; for quadruplets, one in**

650,000 births; and giving births to quintuplets occurs once in every 57 million births.

**38. There are actually more male babies conceived than female babies, but more female babies survive to birth, at a ratio of 105 males to 106 females.**

\* One interesting reason that more male babies are conceived is simply because the "male" sperm (the one with the XY chromosomes in it) is actually *lighter* than the "female" sperm (XX) and can travel faster in search of the elusive egg.

**39. The human gestation period (the period from fertilization of the ovum to delivery) is 40 weeks, or 280 days. Only one birth in 20 actually arrives on the due date predicted by the doctor however.**

\* An opossum's gestation period can be a little as 12 *days*, while that of an elephant can last for up to two years (I've heard that they tend to get a little cranky during the 7th and 8th trimester—ha-ha). If the two-year thing elicited a groan; the Alpine Black Salamander can carry its babies for up to *three* years before delivery (depending on the weather, as it turns out).

**40. There are 247 children born *per minute* in this world. Although deaths occur at an alarming rate also, at the end of the average day, there are 200,000 more people in the world than there were the day before.**

**41. Only horses and humans have hymens (look it up) as far as we know.**

**42. Since 1830, the average age for the start of menstruation (menarche) has decreased by 4 months every decade. . In 1830, the average age of menarche was 16 years while, at present, the average age for American females is 12.5 years**

**43. Humans, dolphins, and the Bonobo chimpanzee are the only animal species that have sex for fun (as far as curious scientists have been able to tell).**

44. It is estimated that 100 million sex acts are performed in the world each day (this may sound like a lot, but it only averages out to 1 out of every 30 mature individuals).

45. The uterus expands 500 times during pregnancy (and the implanted baby, over 10,000 times).

46. During the last 30 years, the sperm count in the average American male has *dropped* an average of 30%! (See: "stress," "environmental factors," the dominance of "stupid-male" TV commercials, etc.)

47. Claiming to "have a headache" to avoid sex (and you know who you are) actually doesn't make much sense because sexual activity significantly increases endorphin production in the brain (especially during orgasm), which has the effect of actually *decreasing* sensitivity to pain in the body (let me know if this one works guys.)

48. Chemical messengers called pheromones are released from human armpits (and other locations) and are detected by other humans, for the most part, unconsciously. These chemicals, even more dramatically than perfumes and after-shave lotions, attract males to females, and vice versa. It has been clinically shown that females even release eggs more frequently (the menstrual cycles shifts slightly) at times when pheromones from the male armpit are plentiful (!).

* Pheromones may also be the reason that women who work or live in close contact with one another frequently find that their menstrual cycles converge.

49. To deliver a baby, a force of 25 pounds of thrust is needed. The uterus is capable of delivering 14 pounds of thrust all by itself. The abdominal and diaphragm muscles generally provide the rest.

50. The hormone FSH (follicle-stimulating hormone) is so powerfully concentrated that a batch weighing less than one *millionth* of an ounce initiates the several powerful events required for the development of mature eggs in the human female.

* One millionth of an ounce is approximately the weight of 1/64 of an inch of a hair on your head.
_____

51. Two months before the birth of a male child, the testicles typically descend from a place within the abdomen, through a small opening in the abdominal wall (inguinal canal), to their final position in the scrotum. If that *doesn't* happen as planned, cryptorchidism ("hidden testicles") can be surgically lowered (or the body will eventually re-absorb them).

52. When a mature human male has a fever, sperm production is temporarily halted (are any of you ladies thinking "bad timing" here?)

53. 15% of couples (who are trying to) conceive during the first month; 60% during the first 6 months, and 80% during the first year.

54. 11% of adults around the world have never had sex (I haven't done the math, but I suspect that only a tiny percentage of them are monks and nuns).

55. In the United States, 4% (one out of 25) admit they were drunk when they lost their virginity (and a few of the remaining 24 still insist that immaculate conception was involved.)

56. Also in the United States, 63% of black males, 53% of black females, 43% of Hispanic females, 48% of Hispanic males, 45% of white males and 41% of white females are no longer virgins by the time they graduate from high school.

* In the United States, about 1,000,000 teenagers will become pregnant this year. 85% of the males that impregnated them will abandon both mother and child.

57. As far as we can determine, only the pilot whale and humans go through menopause. It may not be just a coincidence that in both species, many years are often spent looking after *grandchildren*.

58. Current studies indicate that men who ejaculate more than 21 times per month have a 43% *decreased* incidence of prostate cancer. Ejaculation between 13 and 20 times per month showed an average decrease of 14%. (Propriety precludes further commentary.)

59. Infertility affects 7% of couples who are 30 years old, 33% of those who are 40 years old, and 87% of couples who are 45 years old.

60. The human female breast grows at puberty (cells divide for future milk production, the areola grows, etc.), but they are not considered fully mature until pregnancy, when the breasts undergo a second level of maturation (and I don't even want to think about a third level).

61. It is reported that due to peculiar effects of light transmission through the optic nerve, staring at a blue surface during sex can enhance the intensity of an orgasm (!).

62. The clitoris, with its 8000 nerve endings is almost twice as sensitive (per volume) as the tip (glans) of the penis (to which it is anatomically related).

# The RESPIRATORY SYSTEM

Every cell in your body needs oxygen to go about its daily business of growing, doing its super-specialized thing, and then repairing or replacing itself when needed. When these things happen, like a pile of scrap wood lying next to a newly built home, there are also waste products to dispose of. Not all of the air we breathe is oxygen, and with every breath, our respiratory system extracts the critical oxygen attached to the air molecule and makes it available for distribution to trillions of "hungry" cells. During the second half of every breath, it collects carbon dioxide, one of the by-products of a cell's daily activity, and dumps it back into the environment where hungry plants breathe it in and use it to make their lives happy and productive—and the cellular circle of life continues.

**1. You breathe in and out approximately 20,000 times every day; that's about 8 million breaths per year, for a total 700 million ventilations during the average lifetime.**

\* How many is 700 million? 700 million dollar bills, laid end to end, would circle the earth just about three times.

* 700 million beats of a hummingbird's wings would keep him in the air for almost a year.

**2. During the typical day, you breathe in a trillion particles of dirt and other pollutants. The total over a lifetime amounts to about 40 pounds of the stuff. Thankfully, small hairs (cilia) that line your respiratory tract continually sweep these particles back up into your throat, where they are swallowed (or for a primitive few of you, spit out). Cigarette smoke paralyzes, and then eventually kills these hairs, leading to smoker's cough—and worse.**

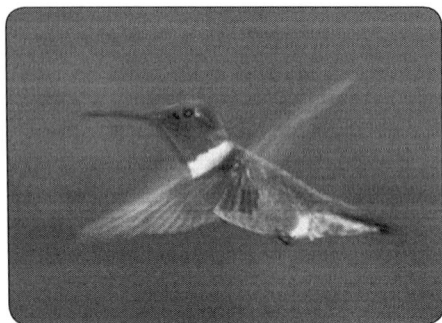

**3. Your left lung is smaller than your right, to make room for your heart.**

* Unless, of course, you are one of those rare individuals (one in 10,000), born with all of your internal organs reversed (inversus viscerum) and salute the flag with your other hand.

**4. At the very far (distal) end of each airway, there are tiny sacs (alveoli) for oxygen/carbon dioxide exchange. You have 400 *million* of them in *each* lung. If these tiny sacs were opened up and spread out, they would cover an area about 100 square meters (1076 square feet), or about 1/3 the size of a tennis court.**

* If alveoli were the size of popped popcorn, 400 million of them would be enough to cover the typical football field to a depth of 3 feet, or almost twice the number of turkeys grown in the United States in 2007.

* It is a little less than the number of BBs it would take to completely fill up 8 Volkswagen "Beetles"; the number of miles in a trip 20,000 times around the earth; and the number of hamburgers consumed in the United States—every 4½ days.

5. Every 24 hours, the average person exhales about one pint of water through the nose and mouth (unless you are a long-winded professor and talk yourself into dehydration on a regular basis).

6. The mechanics of respiration that take place in the lungs (oxygen made available, put into the circulatory system, and then exchanged for carbon dioxide, which is eventually exhaled) occur in an almost identical fashion in each one of the 50-70 trillion individual cells in your body.

7. The process of cellular respiration (gaseous exchange within each body cell), so necessary for our existence, is almost opposite of that which occurs in plants (which utilize carbon dioxide and produce the oxygen and food essential for practically all animal life on this planet).

* It takes 5-7 trees to absorb the carbon dioxide you exhale each day and replace it with oxygen.

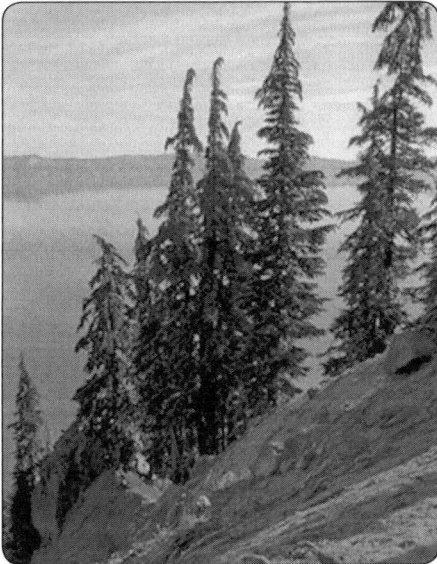

8. Your lungs contain about 1500 *miles* of airways, compacted into a volume comparable to 4 of your fists.

9. Your combined lungs weigh a little more than two small cans of beef stew, and occupy a little more area than two boxes of cake mix. With all of the tubes (bronchioles) and tiny sacs (alveoli), their surface area totals about 50 *times* that of your skin.

10. We take in about 100 billion *trillion* molecules of air with each breath.

* And just how many are a billion trillion anyway? If each molecule were as large as a grain of beach sand, it would be enough sand to fill 20,000,000,000,000,000 (20 quadrillion) cubic FEET of beach (which is actually more beach than there *is* beach along the entire coast of California)—*with each breath!*

* It is a sobering fact that statistically, with every breath, you inhale several molecules of air also previously inhaled and then exhaled by Abraham Lincoln, Moses, Adolf Hitler, your mother-in-law, (or anyone else you care to name).

**11. Each tiny air-exchange sac (alveolus) measures only 1/100 of an inch across, and its walls are only 3 millionths of an inch thick.**

* It would take about 12,000 of these walls, stacked against each other, to equal the thickness of a single piece of paper. For your additional informational enjoyment: if the distance to our own sun were represented by the thickness of that same piece of paper, the distance to the nearest star (Alpha Centauri) would equal a stack 71 *feet* high. Kind of makes you feel a bit lonely, doesn't it?

**12. The gas we exhale contains 100 times more carbon dioxide than the gas we just inhaled (figures vary to some extent, depending on which city you are attempting to breathe in).**

**13. We inhale air that is 21% oxygen, and exhale a gas containing 16%. So we only use about 5% of the oxygen we inhale for respiration within our 70 trillion body cells. That's why C.P.R. (cardio-pulmonary resuscitation) works.**

**14. It's *not* the lack of oxygen that causes you to breathe faster, it's the increase in carbon dioxide level. If you are in an airtight room, you will probably die of carbon dioxide poisoning (build-up) before you die from lack of oxygen (but it'll have the same result).**

**15. During a 24-hour period, a human will breathe an average of 23,040 times, and a total of 420 cubic feet of air (enough to fill about 4½ Volkswagen "Beetles"). During your lifetime, you breathe in enough air to fill almost 10 million balloons (10-13 million cubic feet).**

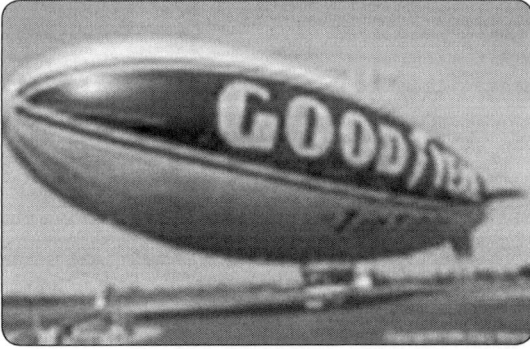

* That amounts to enough air to fill 49 Goodyear Blimps, and almost completely fill the Houston Astrodome.

**16. You burn 14.4 Kcals ("calories") each hour by simply breathing in and out. At that rate, by the end of each day you will have burned 345 Kcals just by breathing.**

* 345 Kcals? That's just about the same amount of energy (also "calories") contained in a medium sized sac of McDonald's French fries.

**17. Normally you breathe only about one pint of air per breath, but your lungs can hold almost 6 times that amount. Of the one pint of air that you *do* breathe in, 1/3 of it idles aimlessly in the windpipe and other air passages.**

**18. The oxygen intake (air ventilated) for a man under 30 years old averages about twice that of a man over 80.**

**19. You need about 60-80 *pounds* of inhaled oxygen per day to supply the needs of your body (at an average of .06 oz per breath).**

* The average room contains about 90 pounds of air in it, but only about 19 pounds of that is oxygen (do things seem a bit stuffy in here?).

**20. The average person can hold his/her breath for one minute. The world record is 17 minutes.**

**21. Almost 50% of Americans snore from time to time, while 25% snore on a regular basis. Almost 20% of you who *do* snore (including those of you who won't admit it) have sleep apnea, a heart-stressing condition in which you stop breathing for periods of 10 seconds or more at a time.**

* Losing 10 pounds of body weight will decrease apnea by a statistical average of 30%.

* Also, those of you who have a neck size of over 17 inches appear to be 50% more prone to sleep apnea than normal "pencil-necked geeks."

*One more disturbing fact: slightly over 1/2 of expectant women snore during their third trimester of pregnancy (lets see the hands of all the husbands who dared to complain—that's what I thought.)

**22. Each of the tiny red blood cells (erythrocytes) in your body can transport 280 *million* molecules of oxygen-carrying hemoglobin. *Each* Hemoglobin molecule carries 4 oxygen molecules to the waiting cells.**

* Let's see how many "players" are involved in keeping our bodies supplied with oxygen. We have in our blood approximately 5 million red blood cells per *cubic milliliter* of blood. Each of these erythrocytes can carry 1 billion oxygen molecules. If there are 3,300,000 cubic millimeters of blood in your body (trust me, there are), then as near as I can tell, that would equal... *whole bunches* of oxygen molecules being delivered to trillions of cells that would die without it.

* Since water only carries 1/100 the amount of oxygen that air does, it takes gills to extract enough oxygen for a human to stay submerged for more than 17 minutes (world record).

**23. Because of the extreme elasticity of the lung tissue, a healthy adult lung is about 100 *times* easier to blow up than a child's balloon (and a child's lung is easier still).**

# THE SKELETAL SYSTEM

In addition to keeping you from collapsing into a heap on the floor, your amazing skeletal system performs a few more critical services. Your bones provide the storage reservoir for the absolutely essential minerals calcium and phosphorus. Keep the bones active by providing exercise and keep the mineral-rich foods coming in, and you probably won't end up being bent over and broken in your old age. And just where do you think your body's 30 *trillion* red blood cells (and others) are manufactured? Right, they're made in the center (marrow) of many of your 206 bones. In addition, your constantly-active skeletal system rides interference for your soft and tender "giblets" when you insist on ramming your body into anything denser than a marshmallow.

1. **Human thigh bones (the femur) are, pound for pound, stronger than concrete. They can support up to a ton of weight (think of a small elephant). We hope you never weigh that much, but it's nice to know that just in case you ever do...)**

2. **The human body contains 206 bones. Over half of them are found in the hands and feet.**

* Even though bereft of fingers and toes, the horse has 18 more bones in its body than we humans do.

3. We are about 1 centimeter (a little under ½ inch) taller in the morning than we are in the evening due to the natural compression of the spinal cord (by gravity/atmospheric pressure).

4. Babies are born without kneecaps. They typically appear when the child is between 2 and 5 years old (The next time you see a baby, go ahead and check, they love the attention).

5. The hardest (densest) bone in the body is the jawbone (mandible) See: "Sampson/Philistines/Jawbone of an ass" (and every day, hundreds of business deals are killed with the same tool- Ha Ha).

6. Your skull is made of 29, mostly fused, bones.

7. We are born with well over 300 "bones", but because of fusion (from cartilage into bone), most of us end up with 206.

8. There are 230 joints in the human body.

9. The bones in children's hands are mostly cartilage. Some of them don't completely change to bone (ossify) until the child approaches puberty.

10. 97% of the living creatures on this planet (the animal biomass) *don't* have a backbone (even excluding wishy-washy humans).

11. The smallest bone in your body (the stapes), located in your ear, is only 1/10 of an inch across (about the same length as a grain of rice).

12. Our skeleton is essentially replaced every 2 years. In fact, *most* of your body is no more than 10 years old. Since birth, the bones in your face have been essentially replaced every 10 years.

13. Bone is one of the few body tissues that continually replenishes itself. When other types of tissue are destroyed, they are typically replaced with scar tissue, but the bone renews *its* damaged tissue— often ending up stronger than it was originally.

14. Bones *start* to form in the human body 9 weeks after conception.

15. Your skeleton weighs about 30 pounds (about 20% of your weight— if you weigh 150 pounds, that is).

16. Approximately ¼ of your skeleton is living tissue (an organic protein called collagen), ½ is composed of inorganic compounds (calcium, phosphorus, and others), and the last ¼ is made up of water.

* To make your bones flexible, and yet steel-like in strength, the collagen and minerals are cemented together, yet the bones in your body weigh only 1/5 as much as comparably sized steel rods.

17. While new bone is being formed in your body (by specialized cells called osteoblasts), old bone material is continually being torn down (again by specialized cells, this time called osteo*clasts*).

*In case you were interested, the fastest growing cells in the animal kingdom are found in the antlers of a moose.

18. Each hand has 29 bones, plus 29 joints, 123 ligaments, 48 nerves, 30 arteries, and 34 muscles (16 in the palm, and 18 running through the forearm.)

19. The bones in your body are not white. They range from beige to light brown in color, and look white in the lab only because they have been cleaned and bleached (or are fake).

20. Once a woman reaches age 30, she begins to lose an average of 1% of her bone mass every year—that's 40% by age 70.

**21. During the act of merely walking from point A to point B, some surfaces on your long leg bone (femur) withstand pressures of up to 1200 pounds per square inch. Being overweight greatly increases the load, strain, and wear.**

* Because of the structure of the joint, an increase of ten pounds in body weight feels like a weight gain of 30 pounds to the knees.

* An Olympic long-jumper's bones may withstand 20,000 pounds (10 tons) of force per square inch on these same joints.

**22. Virtually *all* of the minerals in the body are contained in the bones (99% of the calcium, 88% of the phosphorus, plus copper, cobalt, and other trace elements essential for the body).**

**23. When you were born, you had 33 vertebrae in your spine. Soon, however, 5 fused to form the sacrum, and 4 more fused to form the coccyx, your internal (hopefully) tail. As an adult, you become the proud owner of 26 "official" bones in your vertebral column (spine)— your head sits on the top, and *you* sit on the bottom.**

**24. Without the 1/40 of an ounce of calcium that the bones supply to the bloodstream for continual distribution, all nerve impulses and muscle contractions would suddenly stop, and you would immediately die.**

**25. According to podiatrists, a toddler's feet generally develop better if the child is left barefoot for a month or two after learning to walk.**

**26. During the average lifetime, finger joints will be flexed and extended at least 25 *million* times (especially if you make your living as a secretary...or a writer). Think of it, the back and shoulders may become tired, but the amazing fingers seldom complain about fatigue, do they?**

*If you decided to move your body forward the same distance that only *one* finger moves during a lifetime of flexing and extending, you will have traveled almost 800 miles.

---

**27. Humans have 7 bones (cervical) in the neck. Guess how many a giraffe has. Seven also (but boy, when they get a sore throat….).**

* However, one of the *many* interesting differences between you and the giraffe is that a giraffe can't cough!

---

**28. The spine of infants only begins to develop the curvature found in adults (for "shock absorption") when they begin to crawl. Until then, the spine of an infant is curved like a "C."**

**29. One human in 20 is born with an extra rib (generally males.. hmmmm).**

# THE IMMUNE SYSTEM AND DISEASE

There is a battle going on inside you as we speak (OK, as you read). In fact, there are bunches of them, and they continue 24 hours a day. Sure, we notice and have to deal with the occasional funny red bump on the bumpkis, but potentially life-threatening conflicts are occurring pretty much continually throughout your body. Fairly important skirmishes are happening on your skin, in lumps in your throat and groin, in your bone marrow, sweat glands, internal organs—everywhere, day and night. Happily, the good guys (our immune system) almost always win. Sometimes, however, highly specialized invaders get through our super-defense system and can cause real havoc. We catch a cold or the flu, incubate infections, contract AIDS, develop and even die from cancers, etc.. The vast majority of the time however, if we are healthy enough, we can quickly develop and train specialized defenders of our own—remarkable soldiers who defeat the bad guys and stand ready if they should ever show their evil faces in our bodies again. Eventually, however, if we become too careless, or weak, or are just unlucky—we lose.

**1. The tobacco industry produces 5 _trillion_ cigarettes each year, an average of almost 1000 cigarettes per person on this planet !**

* That's 158,550 cigarettes produced and smoked on earth _every second._

**2. The purpose of the lymphatic system (often called the "second circulatory system") is to wage chemical and physical warfare against invading pathogens (the "bad guys".)**

**3. If your immune system suddenly failed you and the bacteria inside multiplied unchallenged, they would literally fill your body within 48 hours (luckily for funeral people, bacteria fight among themselves almost as much as humans do).**

**4. During a cough, the particles flying out of your mouth travel at up to 60 mph, and those from a sneeze can travel up to 100 mph (unless caught in mid-flight by a thoughtful handkerchief wielder).**

**5. During each minute of every day, an average of 300 million _of_ your body (somatic) cells die and must be replaced.**

* That equals more cells replaced per minute than it would take golf balls to fill up the Goodyear blimp (but only half the number of Twinkies eaten in the U.S. every year).

**6. The tongue is your body's fastest healing part (ironic considering the long-lasting damage it can inflict on others.)**

**7. In many parts of the world, measles is the leading cause of infectious-disease death among children. Because of a simple vaccination however, few deaths occur from this disease in the U.S.**

**8. You have, at this very moment, an average of 100 million bacteria living in your mouth.**

* That's about the same as the number of flies that could be crowded onto a giant piece of fly paper a little larger than the size of a football field—or the population of the United States and Canada _combined._

9. Once detected, it takes about one minute for a white blood cell (leukocyte) to approach and destroy a bacterium. Thousands and thousands of bacteria are regularly intercepted and destroyed as they enter through the skin. If your lymph nodes are swollen, there's a battle going on there too.

10. If you look at it in just the right way (medically), *pus* can actually be a good sign. It is the result of the body's defensive cells eating invading bacteria and stuffing themselves with dead bad guys until they burst.

11. On average, an American dies:
- from drowning every 159 minutes,
- from Melanoma skin cancer every 60 minutes
- from being murdered every 32 minutes,
- from an accident caused by a drunk driver every 31 minutes,
- from a fall every 31 minutes,
- from an accident in the home every 29 minutes,
- from food poisoning every 27 minutes,
- from prostate cancer every 20 minutes,
- from a traffic accident every 13 minutes,
- from complications from Diabetes m. every 13 minutes,
- from breast cancer every 13 minutes,
- from colon cancer every 10 minutes.
- from stroke complications every 3 ½ minutes,
- from any form of cancer every 56 seconds,
- and from heart disease every 35 seconds.

12. In the United States, the risk of dying from
- a mountain lion attack is one in 32,000,000,
- a shark attack is one in 3,700,000,
- a legal execution is one in 3,440,000,
- a snake bite is one in 3,000,000,
- falling out of bed is one in 2,000,000,
- being mauled by a dog is one in 700,000,
- a terrorist attack in a foreign country is one in 650,000,

- ➢ choking on food is one in 370,000 (2,700 per year),
- ➢ from a lightning strike is one in 49,000 (statistically, men are 6 times more likely to be struck by lightning than women),
- ➢ an airline crash is one in 40,000—(even though, at any given moment, 61,000 Americans are airborne),
- ➢ in a tornado is one in 39,000,
- ➢ a fall is one in 20,700,
- ➢ being murdered is one in 18,000,
- ➢ wounds received in an assault is one in 16,400,
- ➢ from intentional self-harm is one in 9,380,
- ➢ catching the Flu is one in 8,000,
- ➢ food poisoning is one in 977,
- ➢ any type of non-vehicular injury is one in 820,
- ➢ injuries received in an automobile accident is one in 88,
- ➢ all kinds of transportation accidents combined is one in 77,
- ➢ and eventually...from coronary heart disease is one in 4.

13. We are saving many more people than ever before. If the world had continued with the same mortality (death) rate that we had in 1900, more than half of the people in the world today wouldn't be alive.

14. The fecal material (rhymes with "soup") of the ever-present dust mites may be the most common trigger for asthma attacks. The average pillow may contain a million of these dead-skin-eating arachnids.

15. The same fungus that causes the odor between your toes (and 90% of the smell in the men's locker room) is the same species that is added to the cheese called Brie to give it its pungent odor (P.S., mushrooms are fungi too).

16. Allergies are a 20th century affliction. The system to combat intestinal parasites that worked so well in centuries past has now overreacted and become over-sensitized, causing the body to respond (histamine response) to hay, pollen, pet dander, and even peanuts.

* When the reaction to the allergy becomes life-threatening, it is called anaphy-laxis.

---

**17. Germs are man's only remaining predator—and occasionally they win. In 1919, the Spanish Flu killed as many people as died in WWI.**

* It is interesting that the medieval origin of the word "influenza" came from the belief that the disease was "influenced" by the sun and stars. It is also curious that the occurrence of many worldwide flu epidemics has had a close correla-tion with sun-spot flair-up activity.

---

**18. During the Civil War, twice as many soldiers died from diseases (408,000) as died from the fighting (210,000).**

**19. A cough can kick bacteria through the air a distance of up to 13 feet.**

*By the way, those electric "fly-zappers" can kick exploded fly parts for about the same distance over your picnic table).

---

**20. The germs in human feces can quickly pass through up to 10 lay-ers of toilet tissue (morals: TP's cheap, don't pick a moment like this to get stingy; and for crying out loud, wash your hands before you serve me that burger).**

**21. According to one study, 33% of shy people suffer from hay fever, while almost no extroverts have the problem (however, statistically, this *could* merely indicate that extroverts tend avoid the country— and that farmers tend to be shy).**

**22. One out of every 100 cells in your body is specialized for defense against disease. If you weigh 100 pounds, one pound of you is de-voted to self-defense. You might not win a fight with Mike Tyson, but immunologically you are a giant (with both ears).**

**23. An average of 32 million bacteria are growing on *each square inch* of your skin (about the same as the population of Canada). That's**

about 100 *billion* of the little guys eking out their tiny existences over your entire body. The population of the entire earth is only 7 billion.

\* How many is only *one* billion? A billion dollar bills, laid end to end, would circle the earth about 4 times.

---

24. Statistically you are more likely to catch the common cold by shaking hands with someone than by kissing that same person (just skip the formalities, I guess).

25. On average, smoking cigarettes cuts a person's life by 11 minutes— *per cigarette.* It is interesting that this is just about the same amount of time it takes to smoke one.

\* It is also interesting that exercising has the opposite effect on lifespan. On average, your lifespan increases by just about the same amount of time that you spend exercising.

---

26. The risk of a female contracting breast cancer:
   ➤ by age 25 is one in 622
   ➤ by age 45 is one in 93
   ➤ by age 55 is one in 33
   ➤ by age 65 is one in 17
   ➤ by age 75 is one in 11
   ➤ by age 85 is one in 9
   ➤ and by age 95 is one in 8

\* By the way, the death rate for men from prostate cancer is only slightly lower than that for breast cancer in women at these same ages.

---

27. The odds that an American woman will develop some form of cancer during her lifetime are one in 3; the odds are that an American man will are one in 2!

28. Diabetes m. is the 4th leading cause of death in the United States. Because of our eating and exercise habits, of all children born in the United States after the year 2000, statistically one in three of them

**will eventually develop Type II (adult onset) diabetes during their lifetime.**

* At present, type 2 diabetes affects 16 *million* people in the United States (about the population of Florida), and is expected to *double* by the year 2025!

**29. "Soldier" cells (Langerhans), produced in the long bones, migrate to the outer skin and "patrol" for foreign invaders (pathogens). When detected, these specialized cells swallow some of the enemy and then race to the lymphatic system "headquarters" and release chemical messages (cytokines) to warn of invaders. "Troops" are then mobilized, which usually succeed in eliminating the invaders.**

**30. One in 15 children under the age of 18 is affected by asthma.**

**31. 50% of the bacteria in your mouth lie on the surface of your tongue.**

**32. Two clinical studies indicate that you can lessen your allergic (histamine) responses to allergens *by laughing* (But be careful, with the sniffing, and flowing tears, this may present a scary picture).**

**33. Statistically, most heart attacks occur between the hours of 8:00 and 9:00 a.m., on Monday! 15% occur getting out of bed, while only 10% occur during sex.**

* One interesting study indicated that among men, of the 10% who died from heart attacks during sex, 85% of them were found to have been cheating on their wives at the time!

**34. Every *day* in the United States, an average of 27,000 people die from some form of heart disease. Half (almost 420,000 per year) die following heart attacks (many of those could have been saved had the symptoms been recognized, and immediate medical help been sought).**

* 420,000—That's about as many as die from all cancers *combined.* More Americans die from heart disease *every year* than have died in all of the wars

the United States has been engaged in since the Civil War—*combined…* and about 10 *times* the number of those who will die in all traffic accidents this year.

**35. Small critters called mites (related to spiders) live out their lifetimes along the base of your eyelashes, (ex: *Demodex folliculorum*) and in your skin's sebaceous (oil) glands. These charmers have between 6 and 16 legs and reproduce while you sleep at night (at the good ol' hotel *Homo Sapiens*).**

**36. All of the bacteria in the human body could fill a soup can. They are so small that a thousand of them can line up in a space no larger than a millimeter (about the thickness of a dime).**

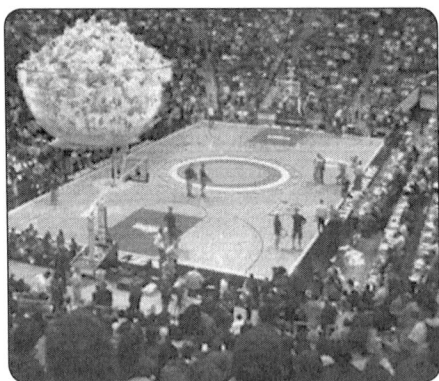

**37. Around 20 million of the cells in your body will have died and been replaced with new cells—** *all while you have been reading this sentence!*

\* If your cells were as large as popped popcorn, 20 million would equal about as much popcorn as it would take to cover the floor of a basketball court to one foot deep—Remember, that's the number of cells that have been replaced while you read this sentence!

**38. A person can expect to breathe in about 40 pounds of pollutants during a lifetime (another source states that the amount is closer to 2 teaspoons *per day*, which the respiratory and digestive systems must eliminate).**

**39. The skin of your armpits can harbor around 500,000 bacteria per square inch, while that of a drier area (such as your forearm) may contain only about 13,000 (close to the average attendance at ice hockey matches this year).**

40. The fibers that cause a wound to clot (fibrin) are activated by a protein (thrombin) so effective that only *one* molecule of it will produce 160 *million* molecules of clotting fiber.

* That would be the equivalent to an event where *one drop* of a substance could pollute all of the water in *an* Olympic-size swimming pool filled 3 feet deep.

___

41. The cells that repair damage to the body (fibroblasts) are so versatile that if they were transported to another area while in the middle of a repair, they would instantly adjust themselves to match the type of skin cell type that now needs replacing. For example, if a fibroblast were transplanted from damaged skin on the finger, to damaged tissue within a knuckle, the fibroblast would immediately turn into a cartilage-making cell (chondroblast).

42. About 100 different strains of bacteria live in your mouth. Almost all of them live on sugar.

43. Some of the bacteria on your skin actually manufacture an antiseptic which kills the bad bacteria that would harm us if allowed to flourish there (which may be a good reason to *not* overuse antibacterial soaps).

44. You kill germs by gargling with salt water (or pouring it on a wound—ouch!) because salt water actually has less water in it than plain water, and as it turns out, less water than in the bodies of the germs. So the water in the thin-walled germs is literally sucked out of the little guy—and it dies.

45. If you find yourself having to fight off an infection or disease, in the time it takes you to read this sentence, *billions* of antibodies will have done their job in defeating pathogens, and been replaced with "reinforcements" to continue the battle. If this amazing mechanism were not in place, you would have died from *any* infection that came along, long ago.

46. The liver is the body's great detoxifier. If some of the things that we put into our bodies (caffeine and nicotine, for example) were to suddenly skip the 6-10 seconds it takes them to pass through the liver, we would die from their poisonous effects in minutes.

47. The 10 million red blood cells that die each *second* after performing their oxygen-carrying jobs must be disposed of. This is accomplished very efficiently by the liver and spleen. Efficiently because the break-down products are used again (actually over and over) to produce more red blood cells as well as bile, which the digestive system uses to break down fats. How's that for recycling?

48. Disease or trauma can destroy up to 85% of the liver's cells, yet it can still function. More amazing still: within a few months after a cure is found for the liver's injury or disease, new cells quickly reproduce to replace the lost ones, and the liver will grow back to its original size.

49. In prehistoric times, anthropoids only lived to an average age of only eighteen years. During the time of Julius Caesar, the average life expectancy was 32 years, and that increased to only 38 years in early America during the 1800s.

\* In the days of Julius Caesar, the entire earth boasted a total population of only 150 million. Today, the earth's population increases by that same number every two years.

50. People who are chronically ill never yawn! When nurses see their sickest patients yawn, they feel it is a good sign of recovery.

51. One in five Americans has genital herpes or some other type of S.T.D. (sexually transmitted disease).

52. The knee is the most easily injured joint on the human body. 1.4 million patients are admitted to U.S. hospitals with knee problems each year (but the most common complaint is a painful back.)

53. The thymus gland plays a critical role in fighting off diseases. It is where your "T" cells (your super germ destroyers) grow up. In children, it is located in front of, and is as large as their hearts. As we get older, it gradually shrinks, until by the time we are 80 years old, it is barely noticeable (One theory is that, as we age and are exposed to more germs, we develop antibodies for them, and this particular aspect of our immune system can afford to shrink).

54. Six out of every 10 Americans don't wash their hands after using the bathroom (my medical students learn to use the paper towel they dried off with to shut off the water *and* open the door—just in case.)

55. Scratching a healing wound site (a *strong* drive), doesn't make sense medically because it tends to irritate the site, which actually slows down the healing process. So why do we do it? A current theory is that scratching may stimulate the release of endorphins, which tends to block some of the pain at the site.

56. A protein in saliva (secretory leocyte protease inhibitor) actually helps wounds to heal. So it might not be such a terrible thing to "lick your wounds" after all (but...considering the quantities and varieties of bacteria in the average human mouth, negative social sanctions, and the risk of contortion mishaps, I usually opt for soap, water, and a Band Aid).

57. If everybody on this planet suddenly decided to remain faithful to one partner, almost all venereal diseases (including AIDS, the fastest growing epidemic in the United States) could be eliminated within two generations.

58. Within limits, fevers are a good thing! As it turns out, they can be far more harmful to invading pathogens than they are to your normal cells, and are the body's natural response to infections and disease.

**59. More people are allergic to cow's milk than any other food. This is due to lactose intolerance, resulting from missing lactase, an enzyme which breaks down that "milk sugar".)**

**60. Over the past 20 years, more Americans died watching scary movies (heart attacks) than died while sky-diving.**

**61. A single organ transplant donor can provide life-altering organs, bones, and tissue, which can save or enhance the lives of over 50 grateful recipients.**

* Please become an organ donor. In the United States, 16 people die each day, waiting for organs that should have been available to them.

# THE **URINARY SYSTEM**

Although some textbooks combine the urinary system with the already overworked reproductive
system (probably due to both the commonalities
in plumbing "exit locations" and medical job descrip-
tions), this amazing system provides us with enough essential services that it really deserves its very own chap-
ter. Every cell in your body goes about its daily business
of building, performing a function, and repairing itself;
but in so doing, they all produce "toxic wastes" which
have to be eliminated—or you simply die. The kidneys,
bladder, and tubules perform this critical elimination
job very efficiently thank you. In addition, the urinary
system is also in charge of the essential business of bal-
ancing body chemistry—24 hours a day. Your two kidneys—the renal organs—are the master chemists of the
body. They not only monitor the quality of your blood
but also maintain the body's internal environment on
other "fronts" by adjusting fluids and mineral levels, including calcium, magnesium, sodium, and potassium.
They do this by reacting to hormonal signals from the
brain and other areas of the body, including the kidneys themselves. It's sort of like an underpaid scientist

by day who moonlights as a garbage collector by night, and it takes an enlightened, forgiving world to embrace the fact that both jobs are essential. OK, a bit dramatic perhaps, but think about this: the best science we have developed so far can offer only a temporary solution for a failed urinary system. It takes the noblest of man's sentiments to come up with a permanent, life-sparing one; the donated kidney.

**1. To be filtered of its impurities, all of the blood in your body flows through the kidneys approximately 40-50 times daily. That's about 45 *gallons* of blood flowing through two organs the size of a small fist—every day.**

*45 gallons would be about *three times* your body weight in filtered blood (if you weigh 120 pounds, that is).

**2. The urinary bladder, when empty, deflates to about the size of a walnut, but can be expanded to hold more than a pint of urine (in children, this typically occurs roughly 10 minutes into your vacation trip).**

**3. Uric acid (the way our body can dispose of the by-product called ammonia without poisoning itself) and is excreted only in the urine of humans—and Dalmatian dogs (both of whom form pesky uric stones).**

**4. The kidneys are about the size of a child's fist; yet the best substitute that medical science can create (the kidney dialysis machine) is only a temporary one. Eventually a transplant of this indispensable organ will be necessary for survival.**

**5. Each kidney contains *one million* microscopic blood filtration units (nephrons).**

* How many is a million? It is the number of pieces of paper in a stack twice as high as the Statue of Liberty or very nearly the number of my favorite pancakes in a stack 4 miles high.

* There are a little less than one million seconds in 11 days, and

* Manhattan Island, tip to tip, is just under one million inches long.

**6. If the tiny tubules in each kidney (which collect the filtered-out urine) were connected together, they would form a tube 50 *miles* long (which you would still need a microscope to see).**

**7. If your urine (rhymes with "wheee") is yellower today than it was yesterday, it simply means that you are more dehydrated today. So drink something! The yellow hue of the urine is generally caused by unfiltered bile in the system (and/or, as it turns out, a diet rich in brewer's yeast).**

**8. During your lifetime, your kidneys produce more than 40,000 liters (8,800 gallons) of urine while filtering over a *million* gallons of your blood.**

* How much is 8,800 gallons of urine? That's enough to fill up the average size tanker truck. By the way, the 8,800 gallons you produce in a lifetime is only 1/100th of the amount of fluid that flowed through, and was filtered out, by your kidneys. The rest was reabsorbed back into your efficient, thirsty body.

**9. The urinary system is so efficient that from all of the blood filtered through each kidney's million funnels per minute, an average of two drops of urine will flow down into the bladder.**

* By the way, the most concentrated urine that we know of is found in the kangaroo rat, which produces only one drop each day.

**10. During your lifetime, you will spend an average total of 6 months sitting on the toilet (although some of you have really kicked up the average all by yourselves—and may be doing so as we "speak").**

**11. In addition to many chemicals, the kidneys precisely control water balance in the body. Why is that important? Too much and the**

body and brain cells can literally drown; too little, they dry out, and death will quickly result.

12. During sleep, urine production typically drops to one-forth that of daylight levels--thank goodness for that.

13. It is said that it is impossible to urinate and give blood at the same time (However, please be sure to ask permission from the kindly Red Cross workers before attempting to prove this wrong).

# AMAZING MISCELLANEOUS
## FACTS

1. The average human body contains enough iron to make a 3" nail, enough sulfur to kill all of the fleas on the average dog, enough carbon to make 900 pencils, enough phosphorus to make 2,200 match heads, enough fat to make 9 bars of soap, and enough water to fill a 10-gallon fish tank.

\* The combined chemistry in our bodies is worth about $20 at any chemical supply shop.

2. Humans cry an average of 17 gallons of tears during a typical lifetime (variables: romance novels, "chick" flicks, allergies, number of children, etc.).

3. The average person (you) manufactures and swallows about one liter of saliva (of various viscosities) every day.

4. One-half of the world's population is under 25 years old (the average age in the United States is 35.3 years).

5. A secretary's left hand does 56% of the typing.

**6.** It takes only 7 pounds of sudden force to rip off a human ear (and about $3500 to reattach it).

**7.** A passionate kiss can burn up to 6.4 calories per minute. At that rate you can lose up to a pound of body fat every year—at only one passionate kiss per day (that is I suppose, if kissing doesn't make you hungry, or for some of you, require chocolate for initiation).

* By the way, 68% of us tilt our head to the right when we kiss, 32%, to the left.

**8.** The average person (it is said) will spend an average total of 2 weeks kissing during his/her lifetime (I did the math, and if that is true, and you live to age 70, that amounts to 47 seconds of kissing every day. Some of you have some catching up to do).

**9.** A person living to age 75 will have slept an average of 220,000 hours (or about 23 years), and about 20% of that time will have been spent dreaming.

**10.** Undertakers report that because of the cumulative effect of all the chemical preservatives we eat, bodies are not decomposing as quickly as they used to.

*Speaking of bodies—In the late 19th century, millions of Egyptian mummies were used as locomotive fuel because they (the bodies) were so plentiful.

**11.** The sound of human snoring can approach that of a jack hammer (85 decibels), and the loudest recorded snore was officially rated at 93 decibels. Sustained exposure to noise above 85 decibels can cause hearing loss (rock concerts frequently exceed 120 decibels).

**12.** The average female uses 6 pounds of lipstick during her lifetime.

* By the way: Many brands of lipstick still contain fish scales—for sheen.

13. 12% of all the people in this world are left handed (that's up about 9% from when we humans started keeping such records). In the 1800s it was estimated that 2500 left-handed people were killed each year using products designed for right-handers.

14. A child born to a mother over age 40 has twice the statistical tendency to end up left-handed.

\* In case you are interested, *all* polar bears are left-pawed (and their skin is black).

———

15. This year alone, 60,000 people will undergo weight-loss surgery in the United States.

16. In one study, 85% of us said that that when we die, we want to die at home (while only 25% of us actually do).

17. Each cell in the human body contains 10,000 times more molecules in it, than the Milky Way Galaxy has stars.

18. Most dreams last a maximum of 45 minutes (although the longest dream tested lasted 3 hours and 8 minutes). Humans dream an average total of one hour and 22 minutes each night.

19. Over the average lifetime, Americans spend:
31½ years eating,
12 years (day and night) at work,
8 years watching television,
2 weeks kissing,
12 years talking, and
6 months in the bathroom.

**We:**
produce 40,000 liters (10,565 gallons) of urine (enough to fill 170 bathtubs),
grow 65 ½ feet of fingernails (about the length of two school busses),
blink 415 million times,
grow 6 feet of hair—just in the nose,
eat 7,500 eggs,
and spend about 6 months waiting for street lights to change.

**20. We also:**
Have sex 3,580 times,
with an average of 5 different people;
have 2 children, and 4 grandchildren,
walk 11,400 miles (about 24 million steps, or three times across the United States—a little less than half way around the world), and
eat 350 pounds of chocolate (the equivalent of 3,733 Hershey candy bars— an average of one per week—for a lifetime).

* F.Y.I., the Danes eat almost three times more chocolate than Americans do.

---

**21.** The average human walks 18,000 steps each day (about 8½ miles), the equivalent of 6 times around the world per lifetime. The average American walks considerably less—about 3000 to 5000 steps per day (the latest advice from health gurus suggests that we set a goal of at least 10.000).

* By the way; With typical stride length, it takes about 2,000 steps to cover a mile.

---

**22.** The average person walks about 4 miles per year just making the bed (assuming that "the average person" bothers to make the bed in the first place).

**23.** Each day the body renews (re-grows) ½ pound of muscle and other body tissues (about the weight of a double burger with everything on it).

**24.** During 20 minutes of exercise you generate enough electricity to light a 60-watt light bulb for 12 hours (assuming that for you, "exercise" means actually "breaking sweat").

**25.** We burn and renew cells so quickly that 20 *million* cells in your body will have died and been replaced *all while you have been reading this sentence* !

* 20 million? That's five times the number of bricks in the Empire State Building, a little under the number of seconds in a year, but less than half the number of hot dogs consumed in the United States *every day.*

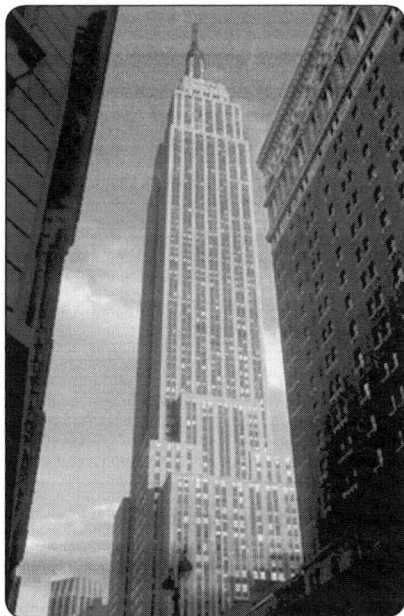

**26.** While for years, right-handed people were thought to outlive their "sinister" (Latin for "left") fellow humans by as much as 5 years, (due to accidents involving tools etc. designed for right-handers) recent studies indicate that handedness has all but disappeared as a determinant of survival (now if they just didn't look so funny writing—just kidding southpaws).

* It is reported that one of the reasons why Leonardo Da Vinci wrote backwards is that, as a "leftie" he didn't want to drag his sleeve through the slow-drying ink.

**27.** One of the reasons that we roll over at night is "nostril fatigue." As one side of the nose grows tired of remaining open and doing all the work, it flops shut, and soon we roll over.

**28.** The average person blinks his/her eyes about 6,200,000 times *per year.*

* If you were to move forward one inch for every time you blinked, at the end of the year you would be *98 miles* from where you started.

**29. In children under age five who lose the tip of their fingers in an accident (up to half of the outermost joint), the finger will spontaneously re-grow. If medical help is used (stitches, for example) the tip will not re-grow.**

**30. There are between 60-80 trillion cells in the adult human body. At 60 trillion, that equals about 10,000 cells for every living human on the earth.**

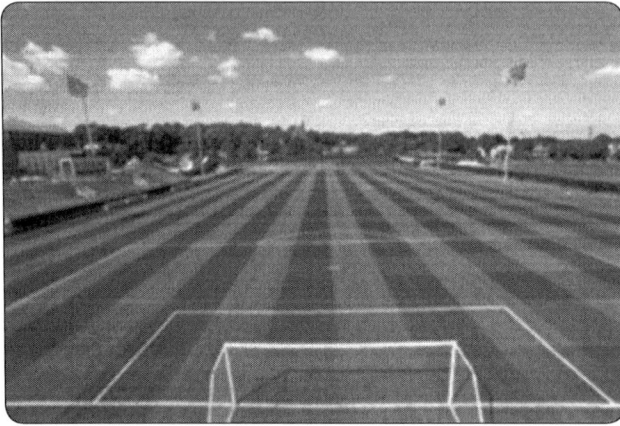

\* By the way: How many is only *one* trillion? One trillion dollar bills, laid end to end, would circle the earth 3,882 times. If each body cell were as large as a BB, only one trillion of them would fill a soccer field to a depth of 25 feet. The weight of all of the humans on the earth just about equals one trillion pounds.

**31. Every year, 98% of the atoms in your body are replaced.**

The estimated 10 to the $28^{th}$ power of atoms that the body contains (or 100,0 00,000,000,000,000,000,000,000,000 of them) is actually more than the number of drops of water in all of the oceans, or grains of sand on all of the earth's beaches!

**32. In the United States, 30.8% of women live to at least 85 years. Fewer than 15% of the men do (but men are catching up in all longevity categories, possibly because smoking rates in men are declining, while those for women are rising nationally).**

\* By the way; Two hundred years ago, almost half of all women died before making it to age 35.

33. Human world records:
>    Shortest adult: Pauline Masters, one foot 9.65 inches
>    Tallest adult: Robert Wadlow, 8 feet 11 inches
>    Lightest adult: Lucia Zerate, 13 pounds at age 20
>    Heaviest adult: Jon Minnion, 1,400 pounds (just slightly lighter than a Volkswagen "beetle")
>    Oldest mother (U.S.): Ruth Kistler, age 57
>    Oldest mother (world): Satyabhama Mahapetra, age 65

34. You can't (and probably shouldn't try to) sneeze with your eyes open (see "vagal response").

35. If we exercise regularly, statistically we add an average of three years to our lives (about the same accumulated that you spend exercising—at one hour per day—from age 1 to age 70).

36. Until babies are 6 months old, they can breathe and swallow at the same time. Adults can't (we call that drowning).

37. The ashes of a cremated person weigh about 9 pounds.

38. When you sneeze, all bodily functions stop temporarily—even the heart skips a beat.

39. The average American speaks about 31,500 words each day (I decided it wouldn't be a good idea to break this down by gender).

40. Worldwide, about 100 people choke to death on ballpoint pens— *every day.* (which is a lot more than choke to death on swords, by the way).

---

* More Americans choke on toothpicks than any other object. Hmmmm

---

41. During the average day at work, the fingers of the average secretary travel a total of 12.6 miles (Notice how thin your secretary's fingers are).

42. The average person falls asleep in 7 minutes (at night that is... figures vary during my lectures).

43. The vestibular organ in your inner ear can detect changes in the position of your head to within the width of a few hairs (see: Special Senses).

44. Over the past 150 years, the average height of humans in industrialized countries has increased by 4 inches.

45. Compared to other ethnicities, Caucasian children are 4 times more likely to be born with webbed fingers (however, this is probably *not* the reason why most of swimming records are held by Caucasians).

46. Afro-American children are 10 times more likely to be born with extra fingers (polydactyly) than Caucasian children.

47. 18% of the U.S. population has sleep-walked at some time in their lives.

48. One in 4 people regularly sneezes when exposed to sudden sunlight.

*I noted recently that in my classes of young medical students, only one in ten knew that you can usually interrupt a sneeze by placing the finger under the nose and pressing inward (just another example of disappearing folklore we apparently haven't passed down to our progeny).

49. Children who were breast-fed as babies have an average I.Q. of 7 points higher than those who were not. (Are there any statistics on mothers who breast-feed their children?).

50. In sleep studies, the human body seems better suited to two 4-hour sleep periods than it is to one 8-hour period.

51. A person can live without food for about a month, but for only about a week without water (and considerably less without air).

52. The body is more sensitive to pain in the late afternoon than at any other time of day (Which tends to make "just wait 'till your father comes home" even more frightening).

53. Human records:
> Most fingers and toes: 14 fingers and 15 toes (on one person)
> Fewest toes: two on each foot
> Most arms and legs: 4 arms and three legs (on the same person)
> Longest tail: one foot long (today, most human tails are removed at birth)
> Longest beard: 17½ feet long
> Longest mustache: 11 feet 11 inches
> Largest feet: size 29½
> Largest nose: 7½ inches;
> Oldest baby tooth removed: 83-year old adult
> Heaviest brain: 5 lb 1 oz (30-year-old man)
> Lightest brain: 1 lb 8 oz (46-year-old man)
> Largest gall bladder: 23 pounds (69 year old woman)

54. By the time the average child finishes crawling, he/she has done so for an average of 93 miles, and all without kneecaps (see: Skeletal System).

55. Humans are the only animals in the world who cry tears (although it's admittedly hard to tell with sad aquatic species).

56. The average person burns more calories sleeping than he/she does watching T.V. (unless Monday night football happens to be on...but then again, if your team lost and you have bad dreams that night..... Ah, statistics).

57. More of the brain is dedicated to controlling the hands than any other part of the body. The thumb is so important to humans that a larger portion of the brain is devoted to using it than to controlling the entire chest and abdomen.

58. Americans use an average of 183 gallons of water per person, per day (drinking, flushing, watering, cooking, showering, making ice cubes, etc.).

59. If you yelled continuously for 8½ years, you would have only produced enough *sound* energy to heat one cup of cocoa (and produced enough bad feelings to alienate many neighbors).

60. There are 4 babies born in the world every second (try to blink your eyes 4 times in one second to get a feel for the world's birth rate). In the United States, babies enter the world at a rate of one child every 7 seconds.

\* By the way, the world's baby production rate per second, is just about the same as the number of cans of Spam consumed in the U.S. per second (led by Hawaii, believe it or not).

61. Every one of the 200 different *types* of cells in your body developed and specialized from just one—the fertilized egg (zygote).

62. There is more water content in the tissue of your bones (25%) than there is in your fat tissue (20%).

63. Your brain has more water content in its gray matter (85%) than you have water in your blood (80%).

64. Worldwide, the average human body has 30 to 40 *billion* fat cells on and in it. (Notice that I refrained from commenting on the effect the average American has on those numbers).

* Interestingly, most of us develop our supply of fat cells during the third semester of pregnancy (no, no, no, I'm not talking about the mother), and for a short period at about one year of age. From that point on, fat cells just expand and contract depending on our ingestion vs. caloric expenditure ratio.

---

**65.** During R.E.M. (rapid eye movement) sleep, our bodies become "paralyzed" because the "body movement center" of the brain is deactivated. That's why we tend *not* to fall out of bed when we have those violent nightmares.

**66.** One human in 200 has eyes of two different colors.

**67.** So you think you're above average eh? Here are some "average" adult American statistics:

|         | Male      | Female    |
|---------|-----------|-----------|
| Height: | 5'9"      | 5'31/2"   |
| Weight: | 172 lbs.  | 143 lbs.  |
| Chest:  | 39"       | 35.9"     |
| Waist:  | 34"       | 29"       |
| Thigh:  | 21"       | 23"       |
| Hips:   | 36"       | 39"       |

**68.** According to scientists with way too much time on their hands, when first removed, human tonsils can bounce higher than a rubber ball of similar size and weight.

**69.** While singing, your amazing vocal cords slam together up to 170 times each second (on a good day, Mariah Carey's can easily double that rate), and travel laterally, more than a mile each hour.

**70.** All of the 220 types of cells in your remarkable body originated from stem cells, which under the influence of DNA, develop into just exactly the type of cell that is needed. However, when a stem cell from, lets say the hip, is transplanted into the heart, it will immediately become a cardiac cell....and nobody knows exactly why or how.

# FUN ANATOMICAL/MEDICAL WORDS

**Bodily functions and Medical situations**

1. Chewing.................................................................mastication
2. Swallowing .........................................................deglutition
3. Burping ...............................................................eructation
4. Stomach Noises................................................borborygmos
5. Passing Gas.........................................................flatulation
6. A Fart..................................................................flatus
7. Stretching ..........................................................pandiculation
8. Nose Picking ......................................................tilexomania
9. Crying Tears.......................................................lacrimation
10. Peeing ...............................................................micturition
11. Pooping.............................................................defecation
12. Has a Fever.......................................................febrile
13. Bloody Nose......................................................epistaxis
14. Lice Infestation................................................pediculosis
15. Joint Stiffness ..................................................ankylosis
16. Baldness ...........................................................alopecia
17. Vomiting...........................................................emesis
18. Itching..............................................................pruritus
19. Using a Stethoscope .......................................auscultation

20. Difficulty Speaking ......................................................dysphasia
21. Difficult Childbirth.....................................................dystocia
22. Hairiness (abnormal) ...............................................hirsute
23. Fast Breathing..........................................................tachypnea
24. No Bladder/Bowel Control .....................................incontinence
25. Making Milk............................................................lactation
26. Difficulty Seeing at Night.......................................nyctalopia
27. Given Birth More Than Once ..................................multipara
28. Inflammation of the Belly Button...........................omphalitis
29. Nail-biting ............................................................. onychophagia
30. Earache .................................................................otalgia
31. Thickness of the Skin..............................................pachyderma
32. Really Thirsty ........................................................polydipsia
33. Fainting ................................................................syncope
34. Runny Nose...........................................................rhinorrhea
35. Dry Skin ...............................................................xeroderma
36. Age-related Decrease in Vision...............................presbyopia
37. Loss of Taste ........................................................ageusia
38. Sneezing................................................................sternutation
39. A hiccup................................................................singultus
40. Winking ...............................................................nictitation

## Bodily Landmarks and Descriptions

1. Tragus.....................fleshy bump at entrance to the ear
2. Frenulum (frenum.............fleshy "tether"—holds tongue down
3. Philtrum.....................indent in upper lip
4. Axilla.....................armpit
5. Umbilicus .....................belly button
6. Lunula .....................moon-shaped curve-base of nails
7. Caruncle.....................fleshy tab—inner corner of the eye
8. Hallux.....................big toe
9. Pollex.....................thumb
10. Glabella .....................flat, triangular area between eyes
11. Antecubital .....................on the inside of the elbow
12. Areola.....................darker ring around the nipple
13. Auricle (pinna).....................outside flap of the ear
14. Vessicle .....................a blister
15. Cicatrix .....................a scar
16. Contusion (eccymosis) ......a bruise
17. Cerumen.....................earwax
18. Nevus .....................mole or birthmark
19. Urticaria.....................hives
20. Uvula......................"hangy-down" thing, roof of mouth
21. Bolus.....................ball—food is formed into, to swallow
22. Vulva.....................female ext. genitalia (medical)
23. Verruca.....................a wart
24. Chyme.....................food which is being digested
25. Lanugo.....................downy hair—covers baby pre-birth
26. Vellus.....................soft hairs—covers you until puberty
27. Vernix .....................fatty substance— covers baby at birth
28. Piebald .....................having a white streak in your hair

## Mostly Medically Related Fears

1. Taking a bath ............................................................ abutophobia
2. Itching ..................................................................... acarophobia
3. Fainting ................................................................... asthenophobia
4. Peanut butter stuck to the roof of your mouth   arachibutyrophobia
5. Muscular un-coordination ...................................... ataxiophobia
6. Being dirty ............................................................. automysophobia
7. Microbes/dirt/germs ................................................ bacilliophobia & mispohobia
8. Body smells ............................................................ bromidrosdiphobia
9. Hair ........................................................................ chaetophobia
10. Food ...................................................................... cibophobia
11. Feces ..................................................................... coprophobia
12. Painful bowel movements ...................................... defacaloesiophobia
13. Insanity ................................................................. dementophobia
14. Dizziness ............................................................... dinophobia
15. Undressing in front of someone .......................... dishabilophobia
16. Vomiting ............................................................... emetophobia
17. Nosebleeds ........................................................... epistaxiophobia
18. Blushing ............................................................... ereuthrophobia
19. Female genitalia .................................................... eurotophobia
20. Nudity .................................................................. gymnophobia
21. Blood .................................................................... hemophobia
22. Doctors ................................................................. iatrophobia
23. Erections .............................................................. ithyphallophobia
24. Loud noises............................................................ ligyrophobia
25. Childbirth (also see #24) ...................................... locklophobia & tocophobia
26. Love making .......................................................... malaxophobia & sarmassophobia
27. Menstruation ........................................................ menophobia

28. Death and/or dying ................................. necrophobia &
thanatophobia
29. Hospitals ................................................ nosocomeopho-
bia
30. Dental surgery ....................................... odontophobia
31. Being stared at ...................................... ophthalmopho-
bia
32. Disease ................................................... pathophobia
33. Children ................................................. pedophobia
34. Kissing ................................................... philemaphobia
35. Beards ................................................... pogonophobia
36. Rectums ................................................ proctophobia
37. X-rays ................................................... radiophobia
38. Defecation ............................................. rhypophobia
39. Getting wrinkles ................................................ rhytiphobia
40. Left-handedness .............................................. sinistrophobia
41. Being buried alive ............................................ taphephobia
42. Injury .......................................................... tramatophobia
43. Injections ..................................................... trypanophobia
44. Urine .......................................................... urophobia

1844942

Made in the USA